Breast MRI
A Case-Based Approach

Caren E. Greenstein, MD
Director, Women's Imaging
Stamford Radiology Associates
Co-Director, Women's Breast Center
Stamford Hospital Regional Center for Health
Department of Radiology
The Stamford Hospital Regional Center of Health
Stamford, Connecticut

Donna-Marie E. Manasseh, MD, FACS
Chief, Division of Breast Surgery
Co-Director, Women's Breast Center
Stamford Hospital Regional Center of Health
Department of Surgery
The Stamford Hospital Regional Center of Health
Stamford, Connecticut

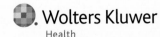 Wolters Kluwer | Lippincott Williams & Wilkins
Health

Philadelphia • Baltimore • New York • London
Buenos Aires • Hong Kong • Sydney • Tokyo

Acquisitions Editor: Charles W. Mitchell
Product Manager: Ryan Shaw
Vendor Manager: Bridgett Dougherty
Senior Manufacturing Manager: Benjamin Rivera
Senior Marketing Manager: Angela Panetta
Design Coordinator: Teresa Mallon
Production Service: Aptara, Inc.

Printed in China

Library of Congress Cataloging-in-Publication Data
[978-1-6091-3236-1]
[1-60913-236-X]
CIP data available upon request

Care has been taken to confirm the accuracy of the information presented and to describe generally accepted practices.
However, the authors, editors, and publisher are not responsible for errors or omissions or for any consequences from
application of the information in this book and make no warranty, expressed or implied, with respect to the currency,
completeness, or accuracy of the contents of the publication. Application of the information in a particular situation
remains the professional responsibility of the practitioner.

The authors, editors, and publisher have exerted every effort to ensure that drug selection and dosage set forth in this
text are in accordance with current recommendations and practice at the time of publication. However, in view of ongoing
research, changes in government regulations, and the constant flow of information relating to drug therapy and drug reac-
tions, the reader is urged to check the package insert for each drug for any change in indications and dosage and for
added warnings and precautions. This is particularly important when the recommended agent is a new or infrequently
employed drug.

Some drugs and medical devices presented in the publication have Food and Drug Administration (FDA) clearance for
limited use in restricted research settings. It is the responsibility of the health care providers to ascertain the FDA status of
each drug or device planned for use in their clinical practice.

To purchase additional copies of this book, call our customer service department at (800) 638-3030 or fax orders to (301)
223-2320. International customers should call (301) 223-2300.

Visit Lippincott Williams & Wilkins on the Internet: at LWW.com. Lippincott Williams & Wilkins customer service representatives are available from 8:30 am to 6 pm, EST.

10 9 8 7 6 5 4 3 2 1

First and foremost, I wish to dedicate this book to all of our patients at the
Tully Women's Breast Center of Stamford Hospital; for them, we continue to strive for
earlier detection and more effective treatment of breast cancer.

In addition to all of these brave women, I also dedicate this text to
two amazing, inspiring, and accomplished young men, my sons:
Matthew R. Heiman and Eric J. Heiman

—Caren E. Greenstein

This book is dedicated to my parents, family, and friends for their endless love,
support, and guidance; and to my patients, past, present, and future for their strength and inspiration.

—Donna-Marie E. Manasseh

ACKNOWLEDGMENTS

The material compiled in this text was accrued over approximately 5 years in a large community-based breast center, which is part of an even larger regional medical center. As such, there are *numerous* individuals who have contributed in one way or another to the material published in this book. If any person deserving acknowledgment has been omitted, please accept our sincere apologies for the oversight.

A special acknowledgment goes to Dr. Robert Babkowski, Chairman of Pathology, whose special interest in breast cancer and commitment to providing meticulous radiologic/pathologic correlation has been a key to advancing the quality of breast services offered at our facility. Similarly, we also acknowledge the other members of his top-notch department, including Drs. Raymond Baer, Augusta Podesta, and Bo Xu.

A very special acknowledgment goes to Stamford Hospital's Breast Tumor Board. This incredible team of health care professionals, led by Dr. Frank Masino, meet weekly (almost 52 times each year!) to discuss and plan the care of each and every patient with newly diagnosed breast cancer at our facility. This multidisciplinary team includes radiologists, surgeons, pathologists, medical oncologists, radiation oncologists, plastic surgeons, nurses, geneticists, tumor registry representatives, and so on. These individuals include Drs. Sherman Bull, Sunny D. Mitchell, Paul Weinstein, K.M. Steve Lo, Isidore Tepler, Anne Angevine, Bruce Baron, Neil Cohen, David Passaretti, Philip R. Corvo, Joey Papa, Frank Masino, Sean Dowling, Robert Babkowski, Bo Xu, Augusto Podesta, Kristen Zimmermann, Arthur Rosenstock, Julie Vasile, Salvatore Delprete, and Leif Nordberg, as well as Michele Speer, Elsamma Johnson, Deanna L. Derdelinghen, Marta Torres, Eileen Fredriksen, Erin Ash, Brie Fantini, and Annmarie Kelly-Geraghty.

Another special acknowledgement goes to the excellent breast radiologists who form the team at the breast imaging center, their devotion to providing top-quality screening, diagnostic, and interventional services is greatly appreciated. These include Drs. William Caragol, Kristen Zimmermann, Harvey Hecht, Elizabeth Glass, James McSweeney, Emily Kirschenbaum, and Dena Miller. An additional acknowledgment for their support goes to the remaining members of our professional group (Stamford Radiology Associates), including Drs. Harvey Hecht, Marc Hamet, Michael King, and Ravi Thakur, as well as Melanie Massell and Drs. Denise Pittaro, William Harley, and Howard Liu. We are also fortunate to have many colleagues from surrounding radiology groups who are breast specialists (including Dr. Kelly Harkins and Dr. Steven Cohen), who readily provide feedback and follow-up when patients travel from one facility to the other. Dr Ruth Rosenblatt is not only a colleague, but also an excellent teacher and role model. In addition, a very special acknowledgment goes to Dr. Josef Bieber for his tremendous support and encouragement throughout this project.

An additional acknowledgment goes to the medical community of Stamford Hospital. This fine group of physicians including gynecologists, general practitioners, internists, family practice physicians, surgeons, and so on. While this group of individuals is too numerous to include each by name, we want to acknowledge them for their devotion to providing top-quality, state-of-the-art, academic-level medical care in a community-based setting.

Our nurse navigator Michele Speer also deserves a special acknowledgment for having been such a strong support to our patients before, during, and after their diagnosis. Her 24/7 devotion to the center has truly been a key to its success. In addition, we are fortunate to have three additional excellent and devoted breast center nurses, Susan Macari, Dianne Bankoski, and Joan Haddon, who supervise the care of our patients during their procedures. The expertise and assistance of our nurses is invaluable to our patients and our interventional radiologists.

Our list of acknowledgements also includes the wonderful team of MRI technologists who performed the approximately 10,000 breast MRI exams obtained during the period of time we accrued the material for this book. These technologists give the extra time it takes to do excellent quality work while providing the support these patients often need. This group, led by Roya Ashrafi-Shafigh, includes Aleksandra Perr, Eileen Gencarelli, Mary Kowalczyk, Margaret Murphy, Justina Markovych, Susan Mott, and Patricia Dinneen.

Our acknowledgments also go to our excellent team of mammography technologists, led by Didi Mrnaci and Kathy Oliva, and includes Mary Levinsky, Iole DelTorto, Melanie Dieringer, Cyndee Dimuzio, Linda Docimo, Elourde Joseph, Tina Kovatch, and Tina Zsembik. In addition, our highly skilled breast ultrasound technologists, led by Annie Giandalone, also deserve a special acknowledgment and includes Merissa Franco, Agnes Krystman, Vanessa Mongello, Svetlana Racheva, and Kathryn Siry. Many other individuals in our department assist our patients and physicians every day and include, Marianne Smith, Joshecka Coleman, Joanne Evans, Jessica Guarino, Bill Gubitose, Regina Holley, Pat Klemets, Kiki Middleton, Carmen Padilla, Cindy Petrucci, Juan Rosa, Melvette Ruffin, Casey Brown, Paula Hill, Richard Kovatch, Claudia Tu, Beth Intrieri, Jane Vigilante, Daniel Tweneboah, Sani Sulemana, Kim Fornal, Rebecca Hackenson, and Kelly Ann Davis.

Our procedure technologists deserve special recognition—their incredible skill and expertise makes performing biopsies in our facility a pleasure. This list includes Anne Giandalone, Lana Racheva, Cyndee Dimuzio, Didi Mrnaci, Iole DelTorto, Melanie Dieringer, Tina Zsembik, Roya Ashrafi-Shafigh, Eileen Gencarelli, Aleksandra Perr, Mary Kowalczyk, and Justina Markovych.

Our special acknowledgement goes to the staff at the Women's Breast Center, Surgery Division. The office staff, Maria Giambattista, Ann Rosati, Bridget Cianci, and the clinical staff, Brie Fantini PA-C, Margaret Witt, RN, and Ann Marie Kelly-Geraghty for your timeless efforts toward the success of our practice and this book.

A special acknowledgement to the Department of Surgery, Dr. Timothy Hall, Chairman, for his tireless energy, support, and guidance, as well to the numerous Attending staff, in particular Drs. Sherman Bull, Philip Corvo, Joey Papa, Kevin Miller, Xiang Eric Dong, and Charles Littlejohn, for your support; and to the resident staff, the future is yours.

Also deserving of a special acknowledgment is our MRS (Mammography Reporting System) coordinator, Consuela Hinton, who has become a breast specialist in her own right.

Very special acknowledgments goes to the administrative team at our medical center, who are dedicated to providing top-notch women's health services. These individuals include our radiology administrators Beth Ann Vara, Ernest Cerdena, and David Sack, as well as the heads of our medical center, whose vision and focus on women's health have advanced the quality of care for women in our community: Kathy Silard, Dr. John Rodis, and Brian Grissler.

Our last special acknowledgment goes to my administrative assistant, Heather Ambruso, who spent countless extra hours in the production and editing of this manuscript; her cheerful and tireless assistance was invaluable.

CONTENTS

PURPOSE

This project was begun with the intent on sharing our learning experiences with other individuals and facilities who are starting to integrate breast magnetic resonance imaging (MRI) into their breast imaging and/or surgical practices. We have accumulated more than 1,000 examples of breast carcinomata on MRI and wanted to demonstrate the wide range of appearances of these lesions to radiologists and surgeons who may not have had the opportunity to observe these findings on their own. Using a "case study" format, we will also share our experiences with interventional procedures that are generated by findings on MRI and our experiences with various modalities used for guidance during biopsies and subsequent needle localizations. Furthermore, we will demonstrate how breast MRI has aided in the optimal workup and treatment of our patients and how we have learned to use breast MRI in conjunction with digital mammography and sonography to improve the quality of care and outcomes for our patients.

INDICATIONS

The indications for breast MRI are numerous, and different organizations have issued their approved indications for this exam. These vary slightly from one organization to the next, and within one group over time. A partial list of these indications can be found in Table 1.1:

Table 1.1

The Centers for Medicare/ Medicaid Services (CMS) approved indications for breast MRI include:

- Cases in which diagnosis is inconclusive, even after standard workup
- Evaluation of the postoperative patient when scar tissue cannot be differentiated from tumors
- Patients with positive axillary nodes but no known primary site
- Patients with rupture of a breast implant
- Determination of the extent of disease in patients with known malignancy, before treatment (to ensure confinement to one segment of the breast)

The American Cancer Society (ACS) recommends annual MRI screening for women with:
- BRCA mutation
- First-degree relative of BRCA carrier, but untested
- Lifetime risk ~20% to 25% or greater, as defined by BRCAPRO or other models that are largely dependent on family history
- History of radiation to chest between age 10 and 30 years
- Li-Fraumeni syndrome and first-degree relatives
- Cowden and Bannayan-Riley-Ruvalcaba syndromes and first-degree relatives

ACS considers that there is insufficient evidence to recommend for or against MRI screening (decide whether or not to screen on a case-by-case basis, weighing pros and cons) in women with:
- Lifetime risk of 15% to 20%, as defined by BRCAPRO or other models that are largely dependent on family history
- History of lobular carcinoma in situ or atypical lobular hyperplasia
- Heterogeneously or extremely dense breast on digital mammography
- Personal history of breast cancer, including ductal carcinoma in situ (DCIS)

ACS recommends against MRI screening (based on expert consensus opinion) for women at <15% lifetime risk of breast cancer.

(continued)

Table 1.1 (*continued*)

American College of Radiology recommends MRI be used for:

- An inconclusive workup on digital mammography/sonography
- Determination of the extent of disease in patients with known malignancy
- Monitoring response to neoadjuvant chemotherapy
- Axillary adenopathy with unknown primary
- Suspicious clinical or imaging findings for recurrence
- Evaluating for rupture or cancer detection in patients with implants
- Evaluating for residual disease when there are positive margins after lumpectomy
- High-risk surveillance after genetic counseling

American College of Surgeons recommends:

Consensus statement on the use of breast MRI agrees with the CMS approved the indications previously outlined, but also includes:

- As part of breast cancer screening for patients at high risk of developing breast cancer.
- For the additional evaluation of suspicious clinical findings or imaging results that remain indeterminate after complete mammographic and sonographic evaluations combined with a thorough physical examination.

Food and Drug Administration suggests routine MRI every 3 years to evaluate silicone implants for rupture.

At our breast center, we perform the vast majority of breast MRI exams as either high-risk screening or extent of disease evaluations for newly diagnosed breast cancer. In addition, we perform this exam when there is an unresolved imaging or clinical question, because MRI frequently adds much more information than digital mammography, sonography, and physical exam. Finally, we consider MRI whenever a patient is about to undergo a surgical procedure and may have an undiagnosed breast carcinoma (e.g., when atypia is present on core biopsy, when mammographic findings are highly suspicious, when there are elevated risk factors).

We recommend MRI screening for all patients who meet the 20% lifetime risk benchmark set by the ACS 2007 guidelines. This group includes gene-positive patients as well as patients with strongly positive family history of breast cancer (usually manifesting as two first- or second-degree relatives with breast or ovarian carcinoma, one premenopausal first- or second-degree relative with breast carcinoma, or a male first- or second-degree relative with breast carcinoma). In addition, as these guidelines state, we consider MRI screening for patients in the intermediate-risk category (15% to 20% lifetime risk) on a case-by-case basis. This category mostly comprises patients with history of prior breast cancer, history of atypia or other high-risk lesion on core and/or excisional biopsy, and women with dense breasts.

We also strongly advocate MRI for newly diagnosed breast cancer patients, except when there is a clinical contraindication (i.e., pacemaker, or medical condition so compromised that discovery of synchronous disease would not alter surgical/medical treatment).

Because the amount of information gained by performing MRI is frequently much greater than digital mammography/sonography, we also consider MRI for other types of preoperative workups (unresolved imaging or clinical findings). We do this because it is very upsetting for the surgeon, patient, *and* radiologist to discover a significant abnormality after the fact, when it might have been readily detectible on MRI before surgery. These type of cases are not uncommon, and we uncover an unexpected breast cancer on preoperative workup once every couple of months that otherwise might require reexcision/second visit to the operating room or even go undetected until the following year or years. We have included several examples of these "surprises" in our text.

Finally, we consider MRI for almost all unresolved breast problems, such as BIRADS 0 imaging or unresolved clinical findings (palpable lump, clinically significant nipple discharge, or focal breast pain, etc.). We have even encountered some very unique situations in which MRI has provided critical information that would not otherwise have been discovered (e.g., in two cases in which DCIS was discovered as an incidental finding at reduction mammoplasty, one had a 6 mm invasive carcinoma seen only on MRI, and other had residual high grade DCIS, also seen only on MRI). Without MRI, these hidden abnormalities may have taken years to become obvious on postoperative mammographic/sonographic imaging or on postoperative clinical exam. When all else fails and you are faced with a diagnostic dilemma, always consider breast MRI because it is currently the most sensitive modality for evaluation of breast parenchyma and breast cancer detection.

INTERPRETION

We present our approach to MRI interpretation at the Women's Breast Center at Stamford Hospital.

We obtain the following series using a 1.5 T GE magnet. (We use two magnets at two different facilities) with seven- and eight-channel breast coils. See Table 2.2.

Table 2.2

- Short tau inversion recovery (STIR) (T2 equivalent series): sagittal images, precontrast
- Non-fat-saturated sagittal precontrast T1-weighted series
- Precontrast T1-weighted sagittal series, fat saturated
- Postcontrast T1-weighted × 4 sagittal sequential sets, beginning at 10 seconds after power injection of 15–20 mL of gadolinium, obtained in 2.2-mm sections.
- Sagittal subtraction series, four sets
- Delayed axials, T1 weighted
- Computer-aided design (CAD)/kinetics postprocessing (we use the Dynacad system)

We perform our interventional procedures are performed using our Sentinelle table, which allows access for more posterior lesions.

When we interpret breast MRI, we arrange our series in a consistent order, which helps to expedite the interpretation. If you have different series in different places on your monitor for each case, your interpretation takes a little extra time while your eyes search your screen for corresponding images on other series. Find an arrangement that you prefer and make this your uniform approach.

We place our precontrast and postcontrast series side by side so that searching for areas of enhancement is easiest. Although we rely heavily on the subtracted series, patient motion can render this series useless. In that circumstance, your visual comparison of the pres and posts will be superior. (Fig. 1.1: precontrast; Fig. 1.2: postcontrast with elongated irregular enhancing nodule; Fig. 1.3: subtraction demonstrating same irregular nodule.)

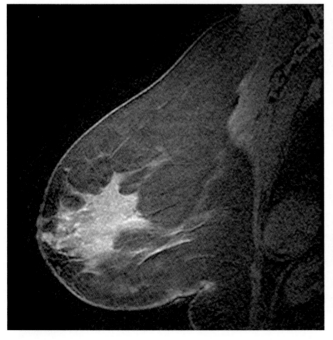

Figure 1.1

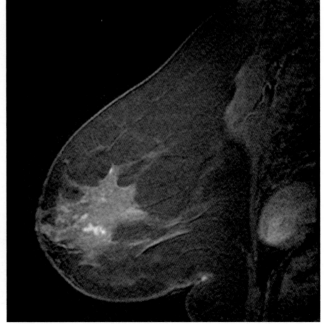

Figure 1.2

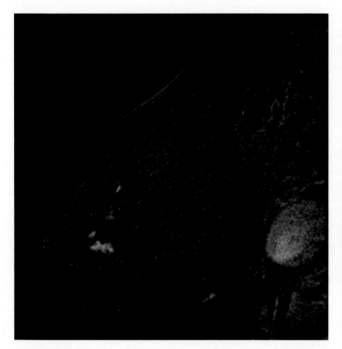

Figure 1.3

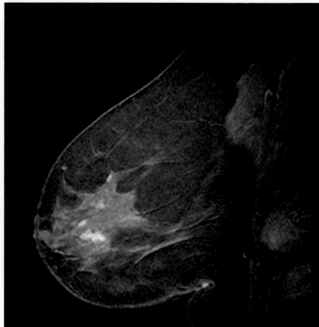

Figure 1.4

When the subtracted images are properly obtained, they are the most important images to examine. Concentrate especially on your first postcontrast or subtraction series (which will highlight lesions with rapid uptake of contrast) (Figs. 1.2 and 1.3) and your last postcontrast or subtraction series (which will highlight lesions with progressive kinetics) (Figs. 1.4 and 1.5). Search the subtracted images *first* to identify areas/lesions of concern. Although we rely heavily on subtraction images during interpretation, the majority of the images displayed in this text are from the postcontrast series, because these are reproduced and displayed more accurately.

The additional series help sort out the lesions of concern, and we use these series to help us categorize enhancing lesions as suspicious, benign, or probably benign. We also use the additional series for comparison with prior exams. A lesion that is enhancing on

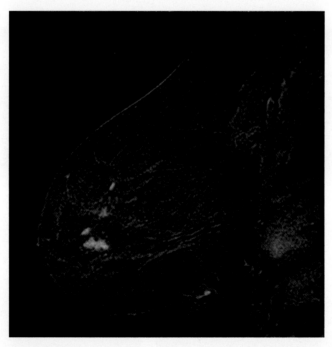

Figure 1.5

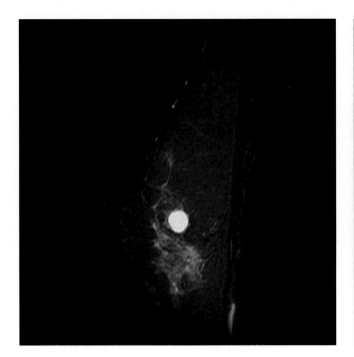

Figure 1.6

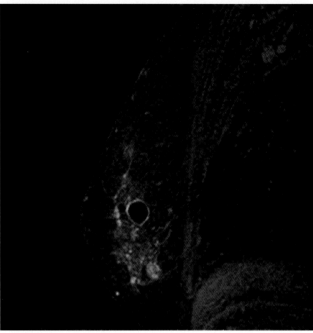

Figure 1.7

the current study (and therefore of concern on the subtraction images) may have been nonenhancing but clearly present and stable in size on another series on an exam performed several years previously.

Lesions that enhance but are very intense on STIR/T2 series are frequently benign. These structures are including benign intramammary lymph nodes and some fibroadenomata. Lymph nodes are typically very intense on STIR images and can be seen to have a characteristic "c" or donut shape. Other lesions that are very high intensity on STIR/T2 series are composed of water/fluid (e.g., cysts, dilated ducts with serous contents, seromas). Some cysts demonstrate thin rim enhancement (Fig. 1.6: STIR series; Fig. 1.7: subtracted series). The inner and outer margins of this rim should be relatively smooth and well-defined. Most postsurgical collections also demonstrate thin rim enhancement. Mucinous/colloid carcinoma can also present as intense lesions on STIR/T2 series. Occasionally, invasive or in situ neoplasm can be somewhat bright on STIR image, so not *all* of these lesions can be discarded from suspicion. Most DCIS, invasive ductal, invasive lobular lesions are not high intensity on sagittal stirs; however, this is not a reliable indicator of benign versus malignant nature. As always, suspicious morphology (spiculated, irregular, microlobulated, indistinct or packaged margin) should prompt further evaluation.

Structures that are high signal on precontrast images contain hemorrhagic or proteinaceous material (e.g., hemorrhage/proteinaceous debris filled cysts [Fig. 1.8], ectatic ducts [Fig. 1.9], or hematomas). Therefore, these structures are also more frequently benign. These also may demonstrate thin smooth rim enhancement. Thick or irregular rim of enhancement suggests inflammation, but rare malignancies can also exhibit this appearance.

Non-fat-suppressed series are of course used to identify fat containing structures. Nearly all fat-containing lesions are benign. We find this series extremely helpful in identifying areas of fat necrosis. The appearance of fat necrosis on postcontrast and subtraction images mimics carcinoma, but when these lesions can be seen to contain fat in the non-fat-suppressed series, they can be safely followed instead of warranting biopsy. Fat necrosis is common after surgery, especially after transverse rectus abdominus myocutaneous flap reconstruction, but also after lumpectomy, reduction mammoplasty, benign biopsy, or trauma. A non-fat-suppressed series is also useful in demonstrating fat or characteristic hilum in lymph nodes (Fig. 1.10), which can occasionally be difficult to distinguish from small cancers because they both enhance and demonstrate washout kinetics. A third usefulness for non-fat-suppressed series is in demonstrating that a palpable abnormality

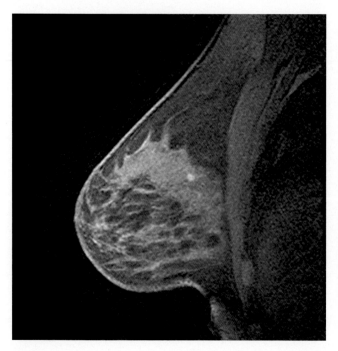

Figure 1.8

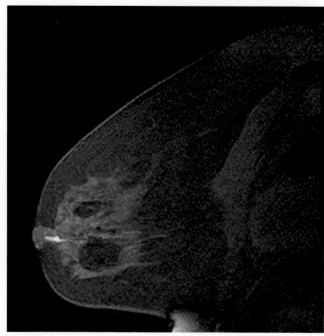

Figure 1.9

represents a lipoma (which contains purely high signal fat within a paper-thin capsule), which can help the surgeon avoid an unnecessary excision.

Delayed axial series are very useful for evaluating the three-dimensional location of lesions, and for comparing location of MRI abnormalities with corresponding cranialcaudal (cc) mammographic views (Fig. 1.11). Axial delayed images may be the best depiction of a progressively enhancing lesion. An enhancing lesion that appears on current images may have enhanced much more slowly on prior exams and therefore been overlooked, but is actually present on older exams. Before calling a smooth enhancing lesion suspicious and recommending biopsy, make sure it was not present on older exams on the delayed/axial series. These lesions can be safely followed, assuming 1 to 2 years stability in size and benign

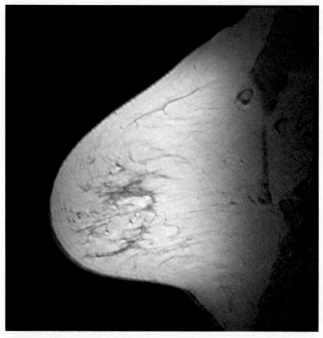

Figure 1.10

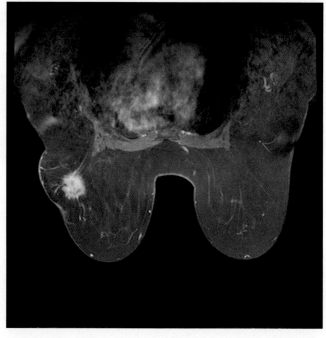

Figure 1.11

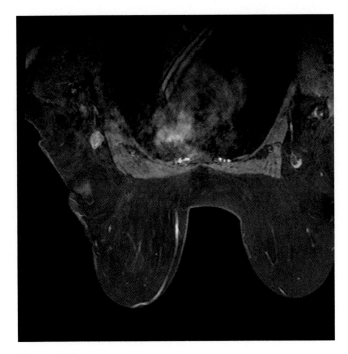

Figure 1.12

margin features can be established, even if the kinetics of the enhancement has somewhat changed. Delayed axial series are also useful for optional visualization of axillary adenopathy (Fig. 1.12). Non-breast ancillary findings (e.g., mediastinal adenopathy, pulmonary/pleural findings, hepatic cysts) can also be more evident on axial series.

For facilities that acquire postcontrast images in an axial plane, merely invert the previously mentioned protocols and evaluate the delayed images and three-dimensional location on the sagittal series.

CAD/kinetic analysis of every breast MRI is performed at our facility. We use the Dynacad system and prefer the evaluation of these data using the visual display (color images) as compared with the graph analysis of kinetic curves. We find the color images give a more readable/observable overall impression of a structures' enhancement kinetics. A graph analysis is done only at the point of the cursor placement; kinetics may vary at different spots within the same lesion. The color display can be adjusted to "fill in" the whole lesion, so the entire lesion's kinetics can be analyzed at one glance. Most carcinomas demonstrate mixed enhancement kinetics, with areas of progressive, plateau, and washout, and appear on color analysis as containing blue (progressive), green (plateau), and yellow areas, in addition to variable amounts of red (washout) areas. Color enhancement maps demonstrate the heterogeneous, variegated growth pattern of carcinomata. Most structures that demonstrate only washout kinetics are actually benign lymph nodes. Only rarely do all portions of a carcinoma demonstrate uniform washout (red) enhancement kinetics.

In our experience, morphology of the lesion has been a more accurate predictor of benign versus malignant nature than kinetics. It is not unusual for malignancies to demonstrate progressive enhancement, especially for low-grade lesions, DCIS, and some invasive lobular carcinomas. The most important role for CAD in *our* day to day practice is in demonstrating homogenous progressive enhancement within a smoothly circumscribed mass, which helps us decide to follow these lesions as opposed to recommending biopsy for them. In other words, we use CAD mainly to support a decision *not* to biopsy a lesion that demonstrates benign morphology. We would never allow enhancement kinetics to dissuade us from recommending biopsy of a lesion with suspicious morphology (e.g., spiculated margin.)

REPORTING

We use Breast Imaging-Reporting and Data System (BI-RADS) reporting for our MRIs because we follow a large high-risk population with annual screening. Our dictations begin with a standard description of our technique (magnet strength, volume of gadolinium injection, series obtained); we also state the indication for the examination (e.g., high-risk screening, extent of disease evaluation, mammographic and for clinical problem solving, follow-up from previous exam). We then state breast density (fatty, mixed, heterogeneously dense, dense) and level of background glandular enhancement (i.e., minimal, mild, moderate, and severe). When appropriate, we indicate the day number of the menstrual cycle on which we are performing the scan. The body of the report describes any pertinent findings. Unless clinically relevant, we do not usually describe in detail any nonenhancing abnormalities. When the patient is undergoing annual high-risk screening, we always make sure that the patient and the clinician are reminded to continue with annual mammographic screening as well because this can be easily overlooked.

Using standard nomenclature, we issue BI-RADS 1 negative, BI-RADS 2 benign, BI-RADS 3 probably benign (<1–2% chance of malignancy; recommend 6-month follow-up), BI-RADS 4 suspicious (recommend biopsy), and BI-RADS 5 highly suspicious (>95% chance of malignancy; recommend biopsy) reports. For extent of disease (E.O.D.) exams, we use BI-RADS 6 known malignancy nomenclature, but make sure that the necessary follow-up (i.e., additional biopsy) is *clearly* indicated and acknowledged by the surgeon and oncologist caring for the patient. We very infrequently use BI-RADS 0 nomenclature, and reserve this only for rare cases that we feel a follow-up ultrasound may alter our opinion of the MRI findings. If we do recommend targeted ultrasound for ultrasound core biopsy; it is imperative that the report be labeled BI-RADS 4 or 5, because the radiologist performing the follow-up breast ultrasound may otherwise underestimate your level of suspicion on the MRI, and nonvisualization of the lesion by ultrasound may result in delayed diagnosis/follow-up.

Using BI-RADS reporting nomenclature allows us to accrue statistics with our digital mammography reporting system. When we review our digital mammography reporting system data for the past 5 years, what becomes evident is that our positive predictive value (PPV) for an MRI biopsy recommendation is as good as or even better than our mammographic PPVs. It does vary slightly between individuals (approximately 19% to 25%), but our overall PPV for MRI biopsy recommendation for the last 5 years is approximately 21%. Because we are now performing nearly 2,000 breast MRIs per year, a substantial portion of our newly diagnosed breast cancers are being detected on MR.

CONTROVERSY

There is ongoing debate in the academic world as to the impact of breast MRI on the diagnosis and treatment of breast cancer. A few centers and individuals maintain the position that breast MRI as an "extent of disease" evaluation for newly diagnosed breast cancer patients entails too much additional testing without proven benefits. Although it is imperative that studies proving the long-term benefit of preoperative MRI eventually become available, this will necessitate many years of data accrual. In the meantime, it is already well documented that approximately 20% to 25% of women undergoing lumpectomy actually have concurrent synchronous disease, and ignoring this fact while we wait for long-term "proof" cannot be considered the safest protocol for treating our patients. Although additional testing (e.g., core biopsy) is frequently performed in the extent of disease analysis, this is a very low-risk procedure that can be performed essentially painlessly and relatively quickly in experienced hands. We do believe that detection of these additional/synchronous lesions at the time of diagnosis allows us to perform the most optimal and thorough treatment for that individual.

The opponents of routine breast MRI for cancer workups also maintain that this examination is elevating the mastectomy rate. Because one of the quality indicators for surgical treatment of breast cancer is a relatively high rate of lumpectomies compared with mastectomy, this is of concern to any breast center. However, one must always keep in mind that, depending on age of diagnosis, anywhere from 10% to 20% or even as high as 25% of breast cancer patients treated with lumpectomy and radiation therapy will develop a recurrence or second primary site of breast cancer within that breast, which will then require mastectomy. When long-term data have accrued, it is hoped and expected that the patients who are found to already have synchronous disease on MRI at the time of initial diagnosis (and undergo mastectomy) will prove to be the same group of patients that would have recurred 5 to 10 years later and subsequently required mastectomy.

In other words, we would expect that overall number of mastectomies would eventually prove to be stable, but the number of patients that undergo first lumpectomy, then recurrence, and finally mastectomy would diminish. In addition, there is a great value that cannot be proven with data: We can avoid the devastating emotional trauma to a breast cancer patient who has already undergone lumpectomy and radiation therapy and then learns several years later that her cancer has "returned." She must revisit the entire experience and now needs a mastectomy. In short, although there is ongoing debate about the long-term impact of breast MRI, one only has to use breast MRI for a short period to realize the huge potential benefits it provides in detection of breast pathology. Now that MRI technology is widely available, trying to stay "blind" to the large amount of additional information you can easily obtain preoperatively certainly seems unwise.

• CASE 1

HISTORY

A 57-year-old woman with family history of a mother diagnosed with breast cancer at age 57. She underwent routine mammogram 6 months prior, which was negative. She had a bilateral magnetic resonance imaging (MRI) for high-risk screening. She is asymptomatic and her physical exam was negative. Her clinical exam was hampered by large breast size.

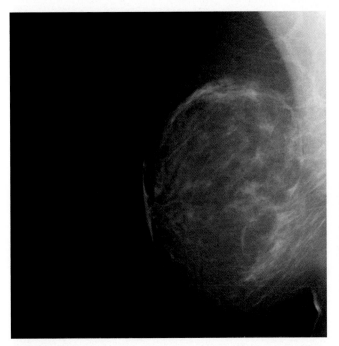

Figure 2.1A

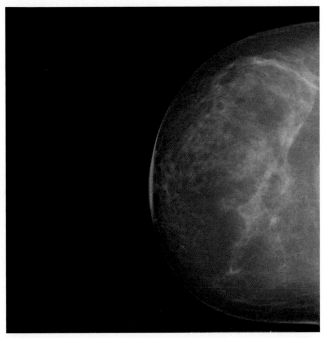

Figure 2.1B

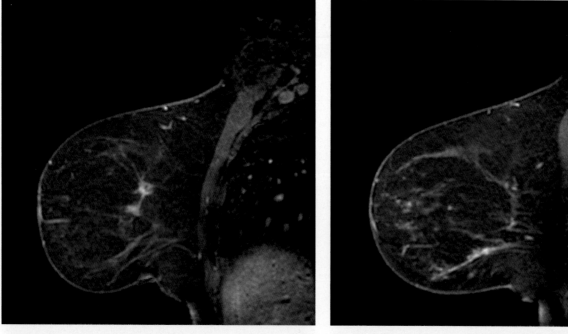

Figure 2.1C

Figure 2.1D

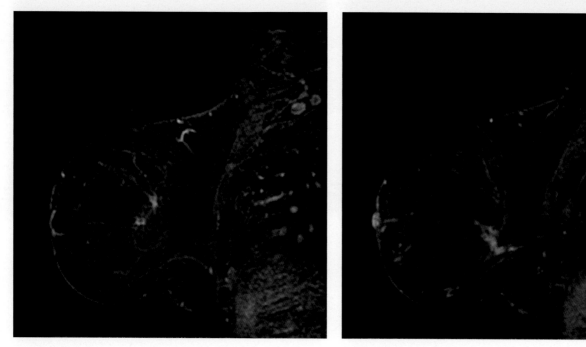

Figure 2.1E

Figure 2.1F

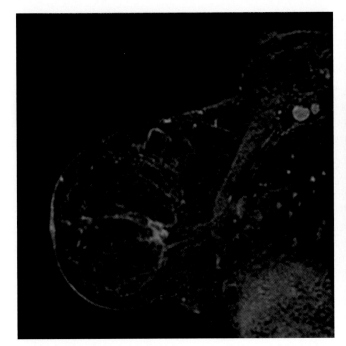

Figure 2.1G

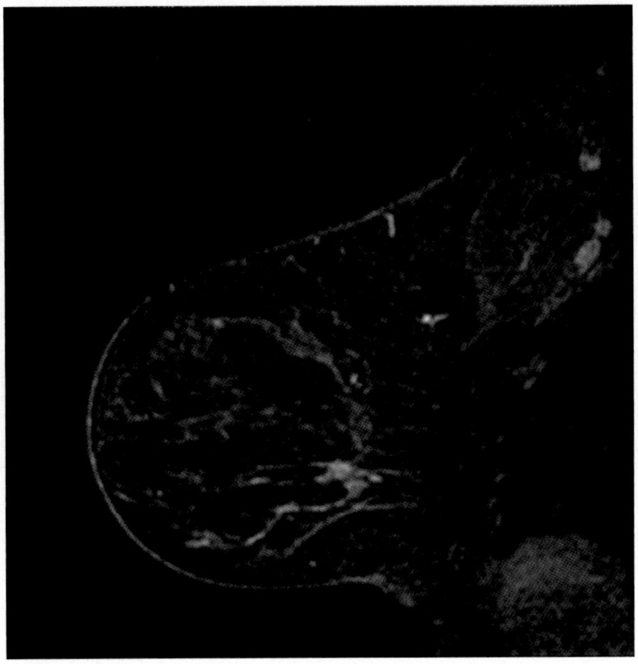

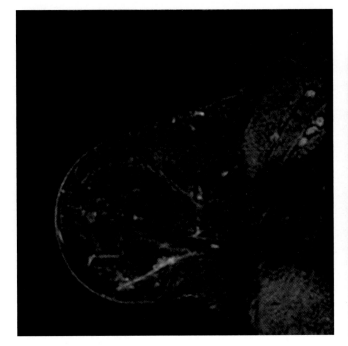

Figure 2.1I

Figure 2.1H

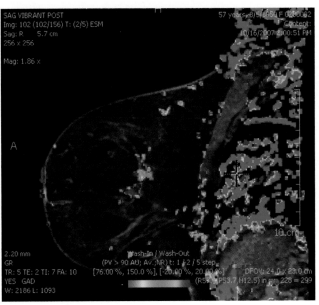

Figure 2.1J

FINDINGS

- Bilateral mammogram—Digital mammography demonstrated the breasts to be composed of mixed fibroglandular and fatty tissue. No masses or suspicious microcalcifications were seen. The architecture was stable as compared with multiple previous exams (Figs. 2.1A–B).

- Breast MRI—The left breast was negative. The right breast demonstrated extensive areas of nodular, spiculated, linear, and clumped enhancement, involving three quadrants, highly suspicious for carcinoma. Also noted was extensive adenopathy, consistent with metastatic disease (Figs. 2.1C–I).

- On retrospective review of prior mammogram, an area of possible distortion was seen to correspond to an area of enhancement in the right inner upper quadrant (RIUQ). This was targeted and stereotactic biopsy was performed.

- Spiculated enhancing areas demonstrate progressive (blue) and plateau (green) kinetics (Fig. 2.1J). A significant percentage of lobular carcinomas fails to demonstrate washout kinetics, so this kind of morphology should always raise your level of suspicion, regardless of the presence or absence or suspicious kinetics.

WORKUP

- A core biopsy was performed and demonstrated infiltrating lobular cancer. Patient opted for bilateral mastectomies and axillary evaluation. On final pathology, right side tumor measured >5 cm, and she had 21 of 36 nodes positive for metastatic disease, Stage 3c. ER and PR positive, HER2 negative. Left mastectomy demonstrated lobular carcinoma in situ.

DISCUSSION

Always review all prior breast imaging studies to help evaluate MRI findings. This will not only add to the accuracy of diagnosis, but may also help in planning for needle biopsy. Although detected on MRI, this was more easily biopsied using stereotactic guidance.

Although this patient did not meet the full criteria (American Cancer Society guidelines) to qualify for high-risk screening, and she did not have dense parenchyma or difficult to interpret mammograms, MRI was very useful in detecting, diagnosing, and characterizing extent of disease.

Digital mammography has a substantial false-negative rate, which can be decreased when interpreted in conjunction with MRI.

• CASE 2

HISTORY

A 59-year-old woman referred for positive family history (mother and father with breast cancer), not gene tested. Asymptomatic, physical exam is negative. She had a bilateral digital mammography/ultrasound (US) and a bilateral screening breast MRI.

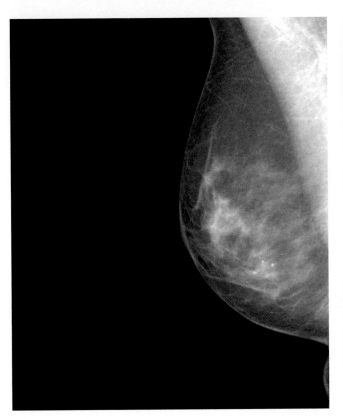

Figure 2.2A

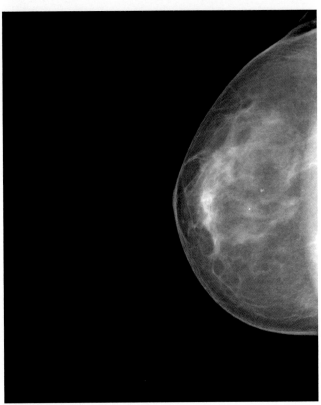

Figure 2.2B

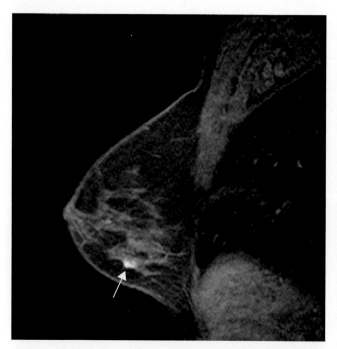

Figure 2.2C

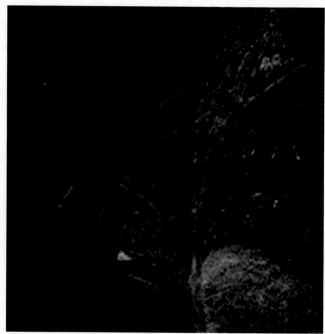

Figure 2.2D

FINDINGS

- Mammogram (Figs. 2.2A–B)—Negative right screening mammogram with stable coarse calcifications; mixed tissue
- Breast MRI (Figs. 2.2C–D)—In the right outer lower quadrant is a suspicious irregular enhancing nodule, measuring approximately 10 mm × 6 mm. Postcontrast series and subtraction series demonstrates an irregular enhancing nodule R breast 6:00.

WORK-UP

- MRI core biopsy was performed. It demonstrated invasive ductal adenocarcinoma. Localization for lumpectomy was performed using mammographic guidance via core biopsy clip. Final pathology revealed infiltrating ductal carcinoma, residual size of 6 mm, sentinel nodes negative.

DISCUSSION

This baseline screening MRI was performed soon after the recommendation of the American Cancer Society for high-risk screening. History of a male relative with breast cancer is associated with very high risk; as a result, high-risk evaluation with MRI screening should be performed.

The breast parenchyma not very dense, but carcinoma is not visible on digital mammography, even in retrospect.

• CASE 3

HISTORY

A 59-year-old woman with a family history of mother and paternal aunt with post-menopausal breast cancer, and a personal history of left breast ductal carcinoma in situ (DCIS) treated with left mastectomy.

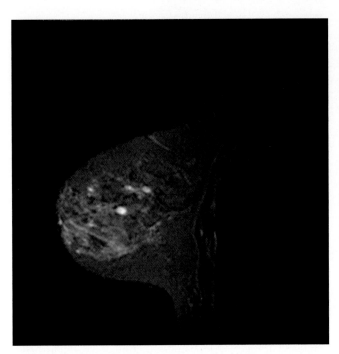

Figure 2.3A

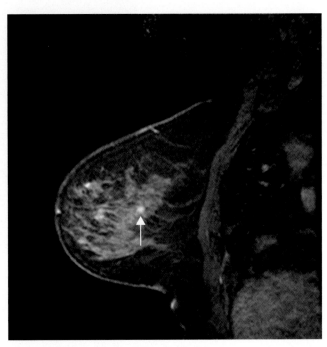

Figure 2.3B

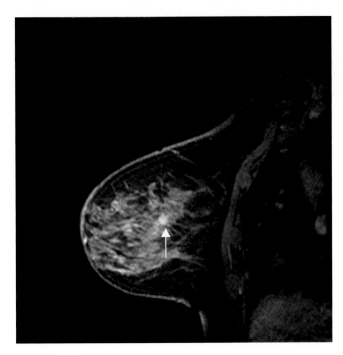

Figure 2.3C

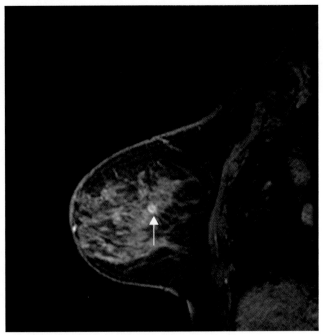

Figure 2.3D

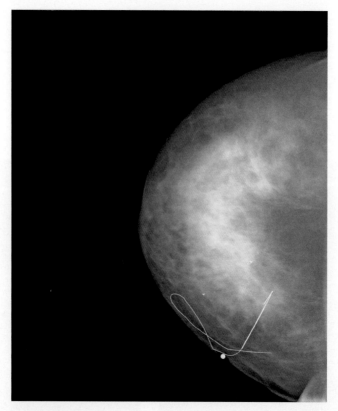

Figure 2.3E

FINDINGS

- Breast MRI (Fig. 2.3A)—Sagittal STIR image demonstrates multiple cysts. Figure 2.3B demonstrates postcontrast, baseline MRI demonstrates numerous enhancing foci, the largest of which measures approximately 4 mm. A 6-month follow-up MRI was recommended (BIRADS 3) (Figs. 2.3C–D). A 6-month follow-up demonstrated focus had increased to 6 mm on first postcontrast series and demonstrates central clearing/ring enhancement on fourth postcontrast series.
- Unilateral mammogram (Figs. 2.3E) —A craniocaudal (CC) view from unilateral mammogram (performed after MRI localization of enhancing lesion showing wire and dense breast), with no corresponding mammographic findings.

WORKUP

- An MRI-guided wire localization was performed at patient request in lieu of core biopsy. Pathology demonstrated invasive and in situ ductal carcinoma measuring 0.8 cm.

DISCUSSION

If there are multiple enhancing foci, but there is a solitary more prominent focus, consider either follow-up or biopsy. The morphologic features, kinetics, and patient risk factors should be considered in determining if biopsy or follow-up should be performed (see Fig. 2.3B—in this image the focus of concern appeared morphologically benign with smooth borders; whereas in Figure 2.3E, the focus of concern has become more irregular and begins to demonstrate suspicious ring enhancement. Ring enhancement is one of the more highly suspicious morphologic features of carcinoma on MRI).

• CASE 4

HISTORY

A 48-year-old woman with history of chest radiation for lymphoma as a young adult. Screening breast digital mammography was negative. She presented for first high-risk screening MRI. She is asymptomatic and physical exam is negative.

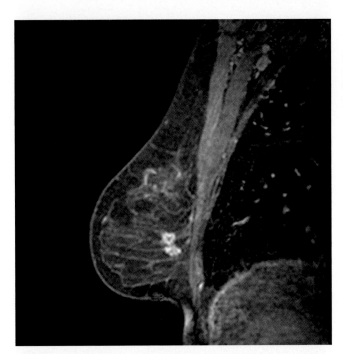

Figure 2.4A

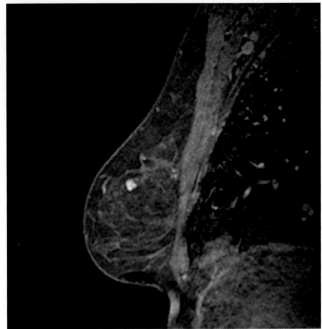

Figure 2.4B

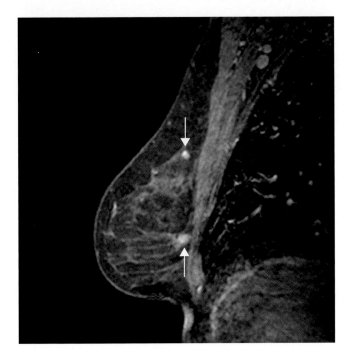

Figure 2.4C

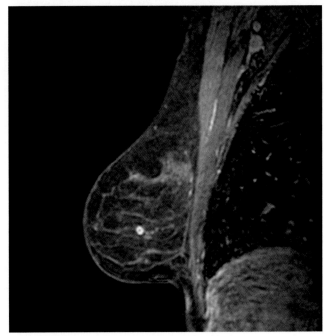

Figure 2.4D

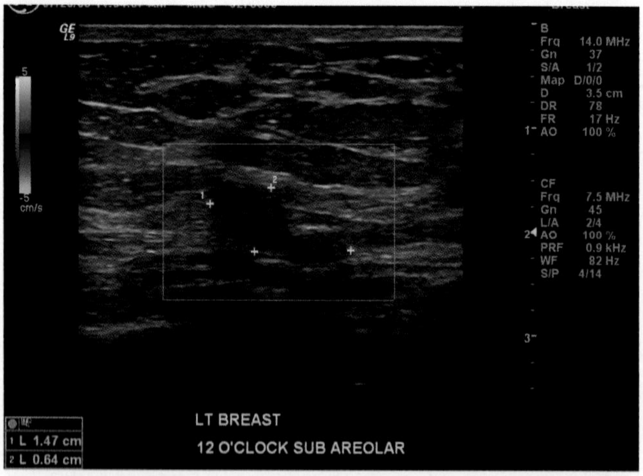

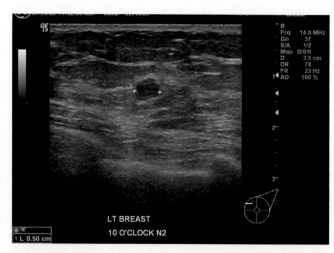

Figure 2.4E

Figure 2.4F

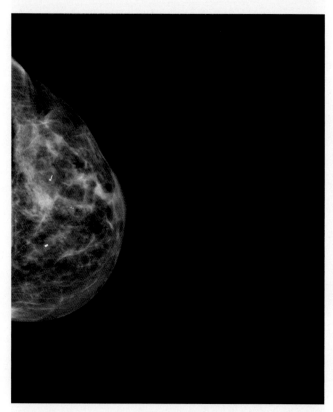

Figure 2.4G

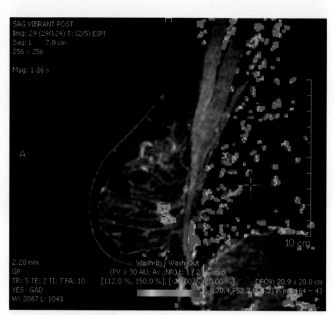

Figure 2.4H

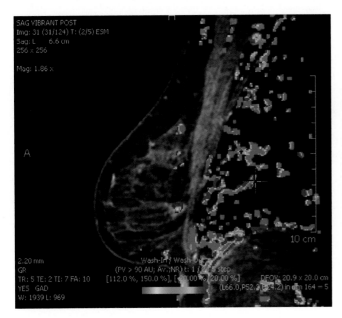

Figure 2.4I

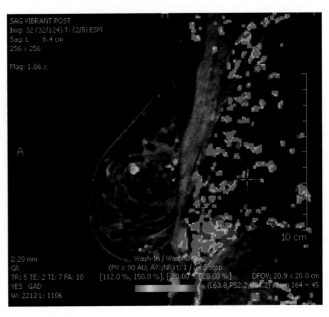

Figure 2.4J

FINDINGS

- Breast MRI (Figs. 2.4A–D)—The MRI demonstrated multiple enhancing nodules (at least four), some of which were smooth and demonstrated progressive kinetics (and nonenhancing internal septation), and others that demonstrated areas of suspicious washout kinetics and ring enhancement. Note the small indeterminate appearing superior nodule.

- Targeted US (Figs. 2.4E–F)—Targeted US was performed and two corresponding, non-specific hypoechoic nodules were identified. The larger area was felt to correspond to adjacent ring enhancing lesions. The smaller nodule is felt to correspond to a smooth progressively enhancing nodule.

- Postprocedure CC view demonstrates two metallic clips and heterogenously dense parenchyma (see Fig. 2.4G) with no mammographic abnormalities.

- Central ring-enhancing lesions demonstrate heterogeneous enhancement kinetics that are predominantly plateau type, but include areas of washout (Fig. 2.04H). This area corresponded to DCIS on final pathology.

- More washout is seen in the superior nodule, which was found to represent an invasive ductal carcinoma (Fig. 2.04I).

- Mixed kinetics, but without washout, are seen in a smooth nodule that was proven to represent a fibroadenoma (Fig. 2.04J). However, we would only assume it to be a fibroadenoma if it demonstrated uniform, homogenous progressive enhancement, had smooth borders, and was smaller than 1 cm in size.

WORKUP

- US-guided core biopsy ×2 was performed. The first area demonstrated DCIS (see Fig. 2.4E); the second demonstrated portions of fibroadenoma (see Fig. 2.4F). She underwent left lumpectomy with wire localizations. The two large adjacent ring enhancing lesions were bracketed under MRI guidance. A third irregular enhancing nodule in a separate quadrant (superiorly) that was not visualized at targeted US was localized and marked with ring clip. The final pathology demonstrated the large enhancing area to represent DCIS. The small irregular superior nodule was a 6-mm low-grade invasive ductal carcinoma. She subsequently underwent bilateral mastectomy with sentinel node biopsies. Pathology demonstrated no residual disease on the left, and right demonstrated atypical hyperplasia.

DISCUSSION

When a cancer identified in one area of the breast, you should increase your level of suspicion of any remaining enhancing areas. Needle biopsy of the second most suspicious area should be performed. If additional needle biopsy is not tolerated by the patient, localization with excisional biopsy at the time of lumpectomy can be performed. A decision for mastectomy should never be based on imaging findings alone without pathology correlation.

Of interest, DCIS can present as a mass with ring enhancement on MRI, instead of the more usual clumped or linear non-mass enhancement.

• CASE 5

HISTORY

A 45-year-old woman, with family history of sister with premenopausal breast cancer, presented with abnormality in the *left* breast seen on outside digital mammography for which a 6-month follow-up was recommended. Her baseline MRI was performed for high risk and further workup of mammographic abnormality. She was asymptomatic and breast exam was negative.

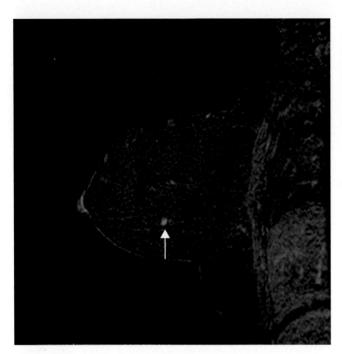

Figure 2.5A

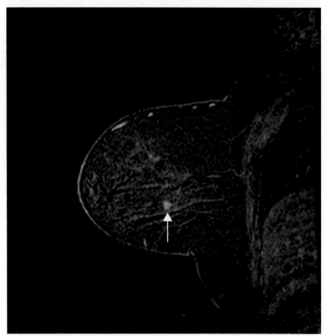

Figure 2.5B

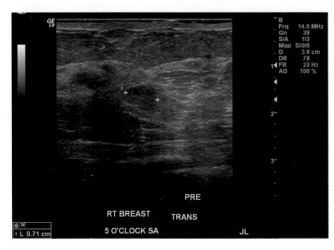

Figure 2.5C

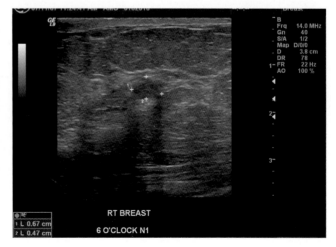

Figure 2.5D

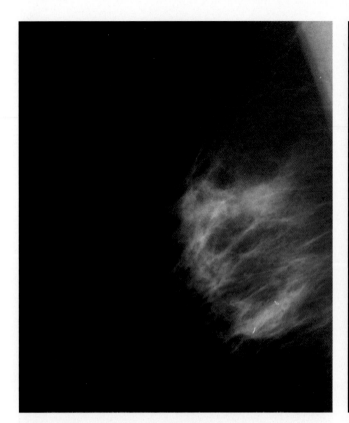

Figure 2.5E

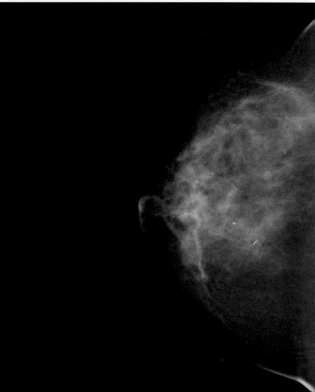

Figure 2.5F

FINDINGS

- Breast MRI (Figs. 2.5A–B)—MRI of left breast was negative. MRI of the *right* breast demonstrated two tiny enhancing nodules in the lower breast (approximately 5–6:00 axis), the larger of which demonstrates a slightly irregular border.

WORKUP

- Targeted US was performed and two tiny nonspecific hypoechoic areas (Figs. 2.5C-D) were identified and biopsied. Pathology demonstrated DCIS. Localization with two wires was performed and demonstrated two separate foci of ductal carcinoma in situ.
- Figures 2.5E–F—Right mammogram demonstrating two clips placed during ultrasound biopsy, no mammographic findings.

DISCUSSION

We perform all breast MRIs as bilateral studies. In this case, it demonstrated a suspicious finding in the opposite breast from the one of concern on digital mammography. We find incidental breast cancers when performing MRI scans for workup of questionable nonrelated mammographic findings, even in women without elevated risk factors.

• CASE 6

HISTORY

An 80-year-old woman with a family history of male breast cancer, as well as a personal history of right breast cancer 14 years previously, which was treated with breast conservation. She had a negative screening mammogram with fatty to mixed fibroglandular tissue, and negative screening US. She was asymptomatic and breast exam was negative. MRI scan was performed as first high-risk screen.

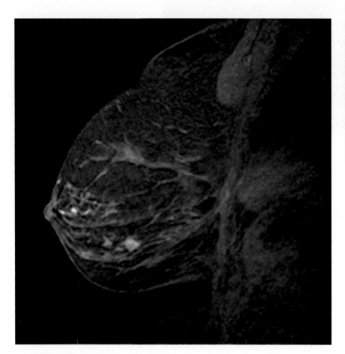

Figure 2.6A

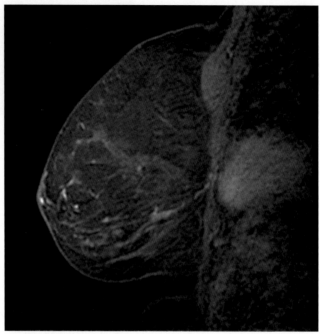

Figure 2.6B

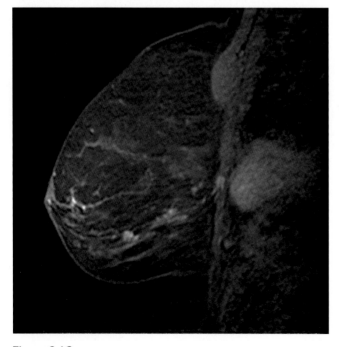

Figure 2.6C

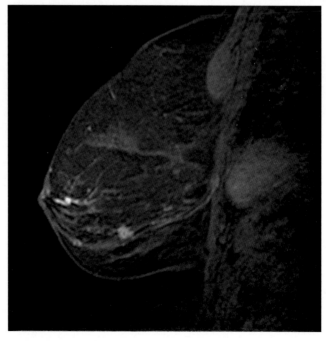

Figure 2.6D

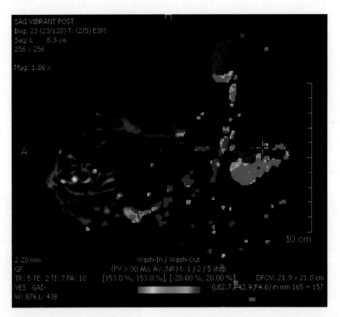

Figure 2.6E

FINDINGS

- Breast MRI (Figs. 2.6A–C)—demonstrates the first postcontrast series with an irregularly enhancing nodule in the 6:00 axis of the left breast, suspicious for carcinoma. Posterior to the nodule is segmental clumped enhancement (seen best in 2.6 B/C) suspicious for associated DCIS. Figure 2.6D is the fourth postcontrast series demonstrating central clearing/ring enhancement at the 6:00 nodule with radiating enhancing spicules. Incidentally noted is hemorrhagic or proteinaceous debris within a slightly ectatic retroareolar duct, present on pre- and postcontrast images, a common benign finding. Color kinetic analysis demonstrates washout in the anterior mass, and progressive kinetics in the posterior segmental region of DCIS (Fig. 2.6E).

WORKUP

- An MRI-guided core biopsy was performed. Pathology demonstrated invasive carcinoma. Breast conservation was attempted with bracketing of the area to include the nearby suspected DCIS as patient declined additional core biopsies. The final pathology demonstrated 6-mm residual invasive ductal carcinoma with surrounding extensive DCIS.

DISCUSSION

Clumped/linear or reticulonodular enhancement near a known carcinoma should be considered suspicious for associated DCIS or satellite disease. If the area is close enough and small enough to be removed while preserving breast cosmesis, this should be bracketed. Otherwise, additional needle biopsy should be performed before surgical treatment. Careful preoperative planning with the surgeon is necessary. The amount of tissue that can be removed while preserving breast cosmesis also depends on the size of the breast, so the decision between lumpectomy and mastectomy takes breast size into account as well.

• Plate 1

HISTORY

A 50-year-old woman with history of contralateral carcinoma with nonspecific clinical symptoms in the right breast. Bilateral mammogram and US were negative. Bilateral MRI demonstrates a 6-mm irregular enhancing nodule in the right upper quadrant. Pathology demonstrated invasive ductal adenocarcinoma (0.8 cm) and three negative sentinel nodes.

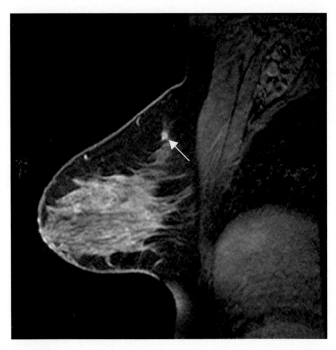

Plate 2.1

DISCUSSION

The lesion demonstrated an irregular margin with mixed enhancement kinetics. In our experience, morphology can be more important than kinetics in estimating level of suspicion. Although this patient did not meet the American Cancer Society criteria for high-risk screening MRI, MRI performed to work up unexplained symptomatology revealed a small carcinoma, which otherwise would not have been discovered in this woman with extremely dense breasts on digital mammography and negative clinical exam.

• Plate 2

HISTORY

A 53-year-old with a family history of sister with premenopausal breast cancer. Routine mammogram demonstrated extremely dense breasts but was otherwise negative. Bilateral US was negative. Bilateral MRI showed a right upper quadrant 7-mm irregular enhancing nodule with mixed enhancement kinetics. MRI core biopsy was performed and demonstrated invasive ductal carcinoma, ER/PR+. Final pathology demonstrated residual a 2-mm invasive carcinoma with four negative sentinel nodes.

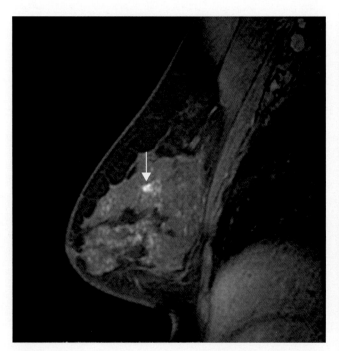

Plate 2.2A

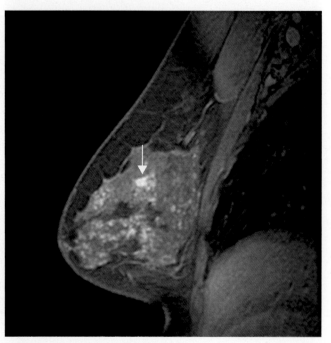

Plate 2.2B

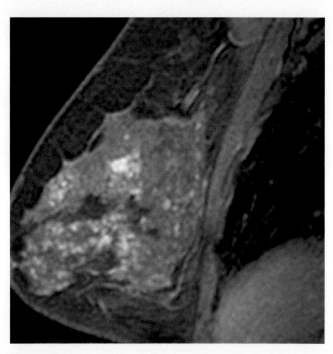

Plate 2.2C

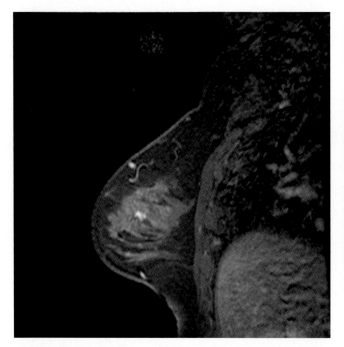

Plate 2.2D

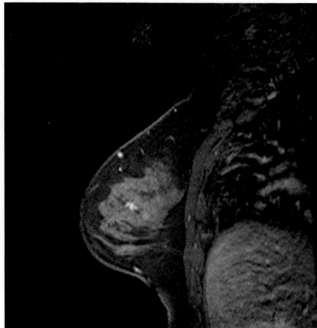

Plate 2.2E

FINDINGS

- Plate 2.2A—First postcontrast series demonstrates marked background enhancement but with a dominant slightly irregular focus in the right upper outer quadrant.

- Plates 2.2B–C—Represents the fourth postcontrast series. Background enhancement has increased, but the irregular focus is seen to represent a discrete 7-mm irregular nodule with central clearing and puckering of the margin. Puckering of the margin is an irregularity that has a similar appearance to a microlobulated mass on digital mammography. On MRI, this is another highly suspicious finding.

- Plates 2.2D–E—Here is another example (different patient) of a carcinoma lesion with puckering of the margin in a 46-year-old woman. Although this enhancing nodule had been stable as compared with prior outside exams (with respect to size), the puckering of the margins and radiating distortion is suspicious and biopsy of this lesion was recommended and performed. Final pathology demonstrated invasive ductal carcinoma (8 mm).

• Plate 3

HISTORY

A 40-year-old woman with family history of a sister with premenopausal breast cancer. She had a bilateral digital mammography, which was negative. Her bilateral MRI demonstrated a new 4 × 5-mm nodule in the right breast with washout kinetics, not visualized on targeted US. Biopsy demonstrated invasive ductal carcinoma.

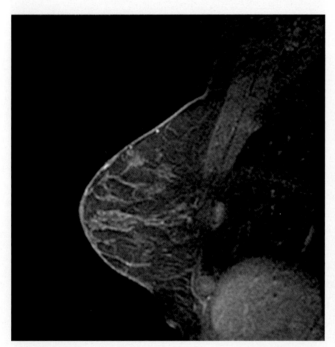

Plate 2.3A

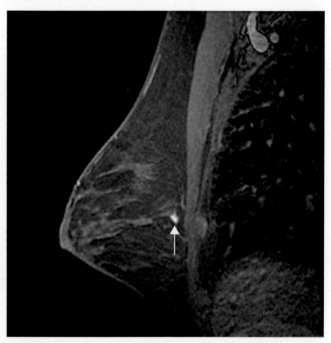

Plate 2.3B

FINDINGS

- Plate 2.3A—Depicts negative sagittal view of the central aspect of the right breast.
- Plate 2.3B—Depicts the same region 1 year later.

DISCUSSION

A new tiny (5-mm) irregular enhancing focus is seen in the posterior aspect of the breast against the chest wall (see Plate 2.3B). Because of its posterior location, MRI localization was performed instead of MRI core biopsy. Grids that allow for more posterior access would make this type of lesion amenable to core biopsy.

Targeted US would be unlikely to demonstrate such a small focus. If it were attempted and yielded a benign result, MRI should be repeated to confirm clip placement in US abnormality actually corresponds to suspicious enhancing area on MRI.

When there is minimal background enhancement, annual MRI in high-risk women is especially helpful in finding these small or posterior lesions, which may be otherwise undetected mammographically and clinically for several years.

• Plate 4

HISTORY

A 43-year-old history of left mastectomy with transverse rectus abdominus myocutaneous flap reconstruction for Stage 3b breast cancer diagnosed at age 38. No family history. MRI follow-up demonstrated new 4.5-mm enhancing focus in the right breast. Pathology: MRI core—DCIS. Final pathology: DCIS.

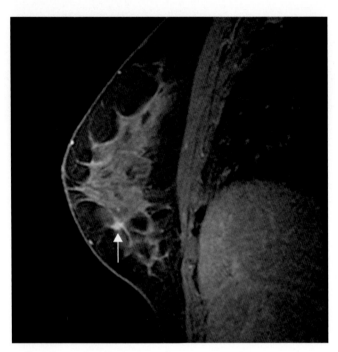

Plate 2.4

FINDINGS

• Plate 2.4—Depicts first postcontrast series.

DISCUSSION

Prior breast MRIs have been negative. A new small spiculated enhancing nodule is seen in the 6:00 axis of the right breast. DCIS may present as linear enhancement, clumped enhancement, segmental enhancement, grouped enhancing foci, or as an enhancing mass (see Chapter 7). DCIS may have areas of washout kinetics but more frequently have plateau or progressive enhancement kinetics. If morphology and kinetics are discordant, we find morphology to be a better predictor of pathology.

• Plate 5

HISTORY

A 45-year-old woman with high-risk screening for strongly positive family history with previous multiple fibroadenomata on US presented for her baseline screening MRI. MRI demonstrated a small irregular enhancing nodule in the right upper quadrant. Pathology demonstrated a 7-mm invasive ductal carcinoma, well differentiated.

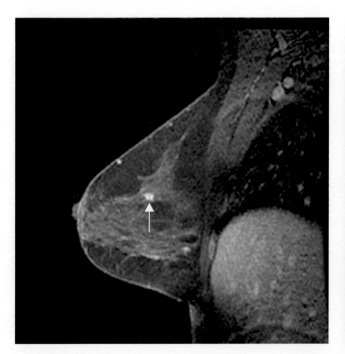

Plate 2.5A

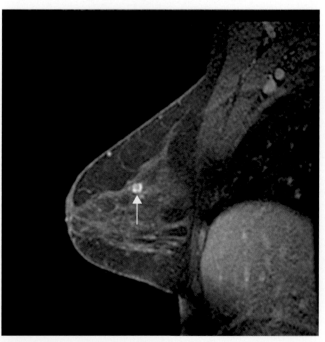

Plate 2.5B

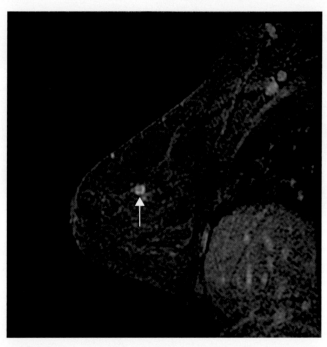

Plate 2.5C

FINDINGS

- Plate 2.5A—This is the first postcontrast series. The enhancing nodule demonstrates irregularity and spiculation of the margins.

- Plate 2.5B—The fourth postcontrast series demonstrates central clearing. Central clearing (ring enhancement) occurs because the central portion of a malignant mass will begin to wash out the contrast on the more delayed post contrast scans. We prefer to use the term *central clearing* when this central washout is only seen on more delayed postcontrast series and use the term *ring enhancement* when this appearance is seen on the first postcontrast series. Central clearing is as ominous a sign of malignancy as ring enhancement, in our experience.

- Plate 2.5C—This is the fourth postcontrast subtraction series. Again, central clearing is evident. Also, the nodule appears slightly larger, which is also a finding that we see more commonly with malignant lesions than with benign ones.

• Plate 6

HISTORY

A 42-year-old woman with a positive family history breast cancer-mother and sister with premenopausal breast cancer-undergoing screening MRI. Her mammogram was negative. Her US demonstrated bilateral cysts. Her MRI demonstrated a 7-mm enhancing nodule in the left breast. MRI core biopsy demonstrated invasive lobular carcinoma, Grade 2, 6 mm. ER/PR+. Final pathology: 1.1 cm invasive lobular with lobular carcinoma in situ and six negative sentinel nodes.

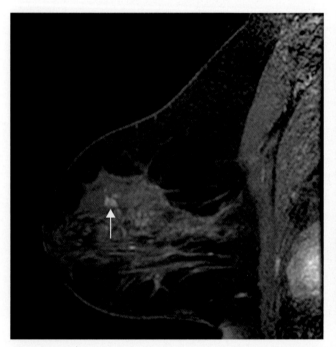 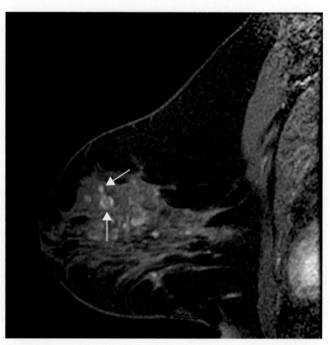

Plate 2.6A   Plate 2.6B

FINDINGS

- Plate 2.6A—The first postcontrast series demonstrates enhancing spiculated nodule with angular margins on background of severe glandular enhancement and numerous small enhancing nodules.
- Plate 2.6B—The fourth postcontrast series demonstrates central clearing of the larger nodule with a second smaller superior satellite nodule becoming more distinct.

DISCUSSION

Background enhancement can limit the sensitivity for detection of small enhancing malignancies. Some use the rule of thumb of ignoring lesions smaller than 5 mm, but with improved resolution and decreased slice thickness, smaller and smaller lesions are becoming detectable. Analyze every lesion the same way you would mammographically when there are multiple findings. Multiplicity and bilaterality favors benign etiology, but if one area appears to have differing morphology (or kinetics) than the others, be more suspicious. Angular, irregular, speculated, or microlobulated margins are suspicions. We sample any suspicious lesions, but may follow a lesion with smooth margins in 6 months. If there is any change at 6 months, biopsy becomes mandatory.

Note also that a lesion may appear larger on more delayed images (i.e, fourth postcontrast series) than on initial imaging (first postcontrast series). The size on the delayed images probably correlates more closely with the final pathology size measurement.

• CASE 1

HISTORY

A 57-year-old woman with a previous history of Stage 0 breast cancer in the right breast treated with lumpectomy and radiation. Her physical exam was unremarkable.

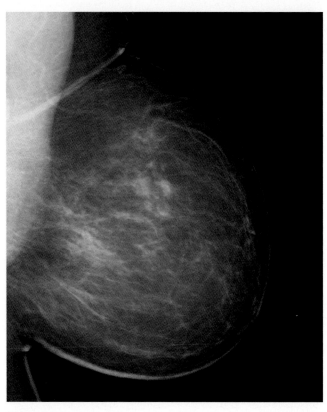

Figure 3.1A

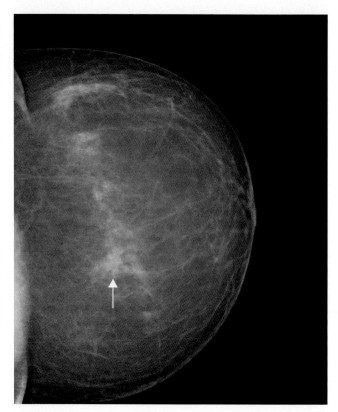

Figure 3.1B

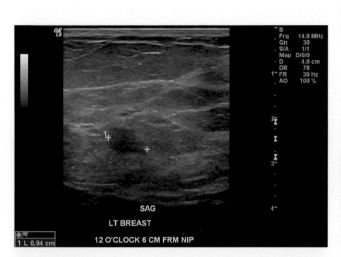

Figure 3.1C

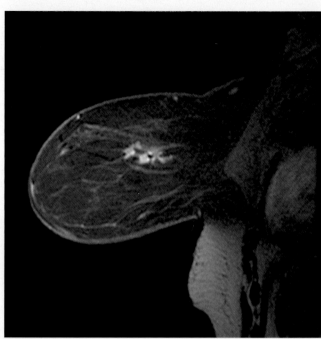

Figure 3.1D

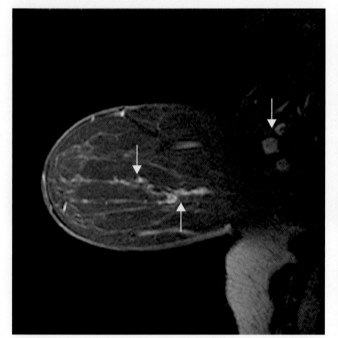

Figure 3.1E

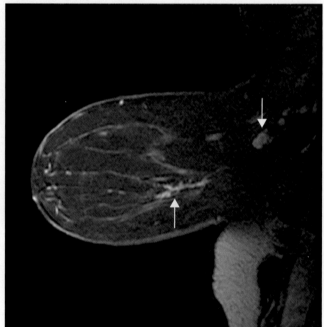

Figure 3.1F

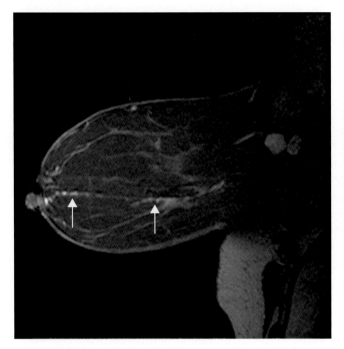

Figure 3.1G

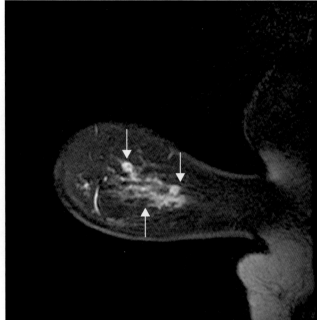

Figure 3.1H

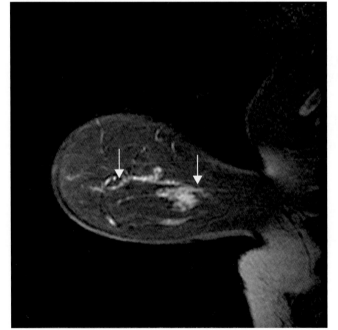

Figure 3.1I

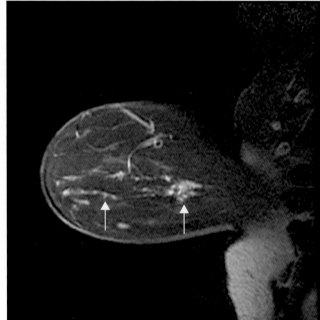

Figure 3.1J

FINDINGS

- Bilateral screening mammogram—1.5 left breast irregular developing density in the 11–12:00 axis (Figs. 3.1A–B), with a corresponding 1.3-cm hypoechoic ultrasound, irregular solid nodule on ultrasound (US) (Fig. 3.1C).

WORKUP

- A US-guided core biopsy was performed and demonstrated invasive ductal carcinoma with high-grade ductal carcinoma in situ (DCIS).
- Breast MRI done for extent of disease evaluation (Figs. 3.1D–J) demonstrates an irregular enhancing mass in the 11–12:00 axis consistent with the index lesion (Fig. 3.1D). In addition there is extensive linear clumped enhancement throughout the lower breast (5–6:00 axis) (Figs. 3.1E–G) extending from the nipple to the posterior third. Multiple additional enhancing nodules and extensive clumped enhancement are also seen in the outer breast (3–4:00 axis) (Figs. 3.1H–J).
- Also noted was adenopathy consistent with metastatic disease (Figs. 3.1E–G).
- Additional magnetic resonance imaging (MRI)-guided biopsy of left outer breast and left anterior (retroareolar) breast confirmed synchronous disease. Fine-needle aspiration biopsy of left axillary node done with US guidance confirmed axillary involvement.
- Mastectomy and axillary dissection were performed. Final pathology demonstrated an upper 2.5-cm invasive ductal cancer with extensive DCIS as well as an inferior invasive tumor (2.0 cm), also with extensive DCIS. Axillary dissection demonstrated 9/31 nodes positive per metastases.

DISCUSSION

Although the patient had fatty breasts on digital mammography and was undergoing careful annual surveillance, she developed almost four quadrant disease and lymph node metastases before mammographic detection. We perform extent of disease evaluation in nearly every newly diagnosed breast carcinoma because additional/synchronous areas of disease may not be detected mammographically, even in fatty breasts.

Unfortunately, this patient was not being screened with MRI because personal history of breast carcinoma does not meet the American Cancer Society criteria for high risk screening.

• CASE 2

HISTORY

A 62-year-old woman had a diagnostic mammogram. Her physical exam was significant for a left palpable density noted in the 2:00 axis.

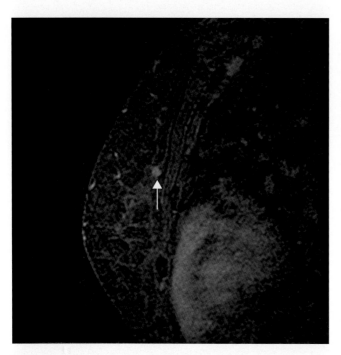

Figure 3.2A

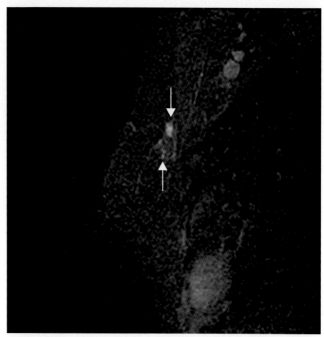

Figure 3.2B

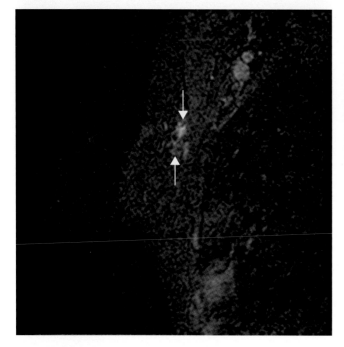

Figure 3.2C

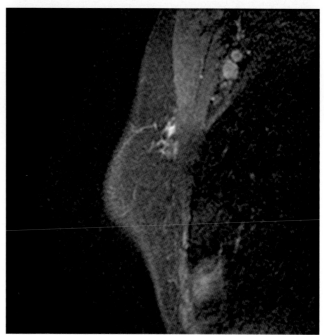

Figure 3.2D

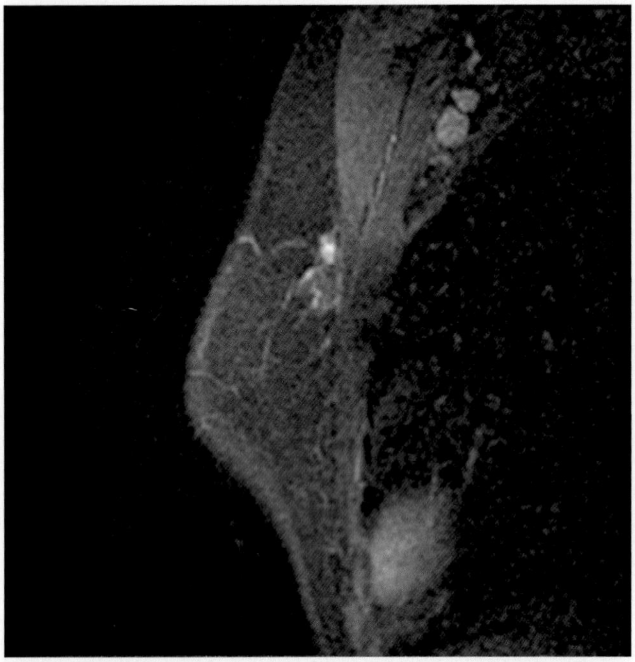

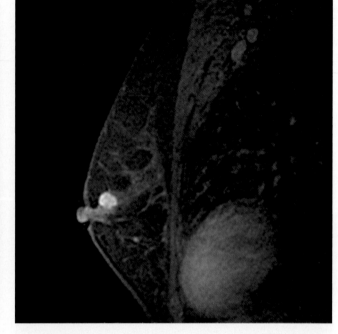

Figure 3.2E

Figure 3.2F

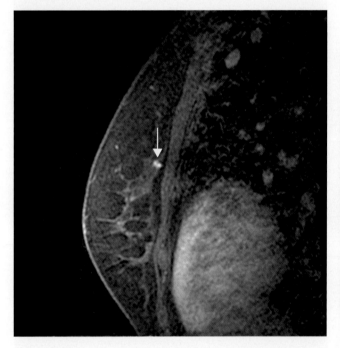

Figure 3.2G

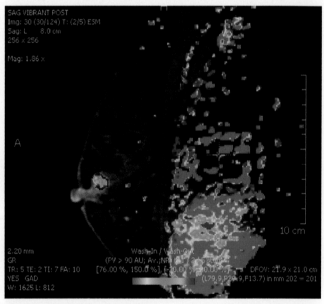

Figure 3.2H

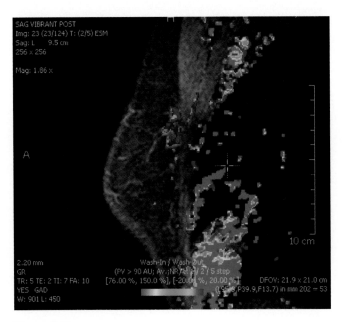

SAG VIBRANT POST
Img: 23 (23/124) T: (2/5) ESM
Sag: L   9.5 cm
256 × 256

Mag: 1.86 ×

A

10 cm

2.20 mm
GR
TR: 5 TE: 2 TI: 7 FA: 10
YES GAD
W: 901 L: 450

Wash-In / Wash-Out
(PV > 90 AU; Av.;NR) 2 / 5 step
[76.00 %, 150.0 %], [-20.00 %, 20.00 %]
DFOV: 21.9 × 21.0 cm
(195 ,P39.9,F13.7) in mm 202 = 53

Figure 3.2I

FINDINGS

- Bilateral mammogram—A new smooth 1-cm mass in the left retroareolar region. This was also identified on US (outside facility). Us-guided core biopsy confirmed the presence of invasive ductal carcinoma.

- She had breast MRI for extent of disease workup. Breast MRI demonstrated the index retroareolar lesion to be a well circumscribed ring enhancing mass (Fig. 3.2H). In addition, there was a subtle area of clumped progressive enhancement in the axillary tail (Figs. 3.2D–G, postcontrast and subtraction images) and an enhancing focus with washout kinetics on the chest wall in the upper inner quadrant (Fig. 3.2C)

- Figures 3.2A–B—Demonstrates mixed enhancement kinetics (which are predominantly plateau but include small areas of washout) in the known retroareolar 1 cm invasive ductal cancer, but mostly progressive enhancement in the large enhancing lesion in the axillary tail, which was later found to represent a 2.2-cm invasive lobular carcinoma.

- Figures 3.2C–H—Breast MRI

WORKUP

- Targeted US core biopsies were performed. At the 2:00 (axillary tail), pathology demonstrated infiltrating lobular carcinoma; at the 10:00 (upper inner quadrant), infiltrating ductal carcinoma.

- She had a left total mastectomy with sentinel node biopsy, retroareolar: 1-cm invasive ductal; 2:00: 2.2-cm invasive lobular; 10:00: 5-mm invasive ductal, lymph node biopsy was positive (1 node).

DISCUSSION

Extent of disease evaluations commonly show unexpected disease that is not seen at all on digital mammography or sonography, or is only seen in retrospect. In our experience, about 20% of breast carcinomas prove to have mammographically/sonographically occult synchronous disease. Whether MRI findings are obviously or questionably malignant, pathology proof is necessary before using the information from MRI to alter patient's surgical management.

When a lesion appears so close to the chest wall that it extends into the fat plane, increase your level of suspicion, as we have found benign lesions to be less likely to give this appearance (Fig. 3.2D).

Even though the axillary tail lesion demonstrated benign (progressive) enhancement kinetics, the morphology and the clinical setting warrant biopsy as opposed to follow-up. In the setting of high-risk screening or extent of disease evaluation, the threshold for making something BIRADS 4 (suspicious, core biopsy) instead of BIRADS 3 (probably benign recc follow-up in 6 months) should be lower.

• CASE 3

HISTORY

A 41-year-old woman 7 months postpartum presents with a physical exam demonstrating a suspicious mass in the left breast in the upper outer quadrant. She has a family history of a mother with premenopausal breast cancer, but was not undergoing MRI screening.

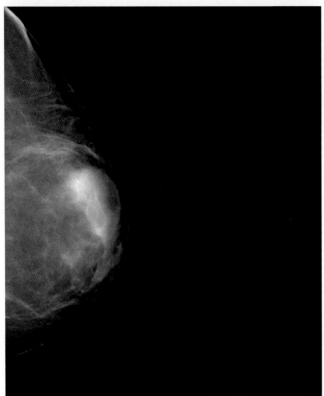

Figure 3.3A

Figure 3.3B

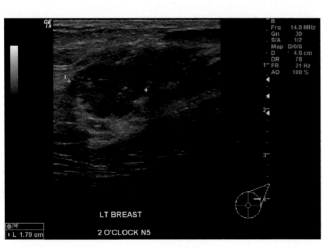

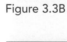

Figure 3.3C

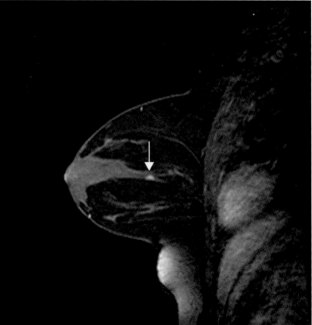

Figure 3.3D

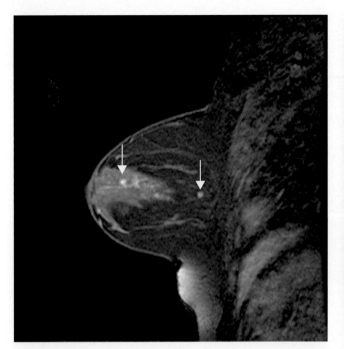

Figure 3.3E

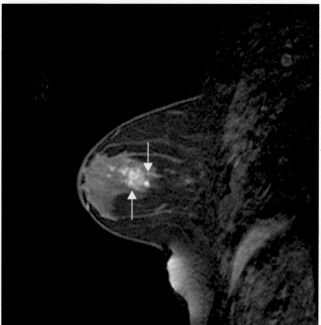

Figure 3.3F

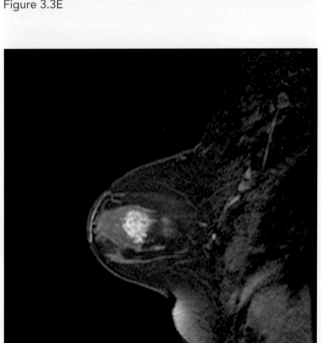

Figure 3.3G

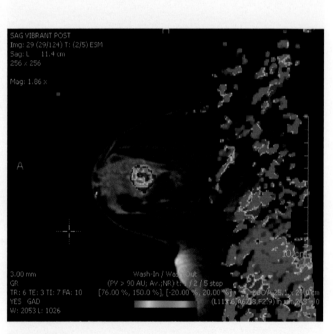

Figure 3.3H

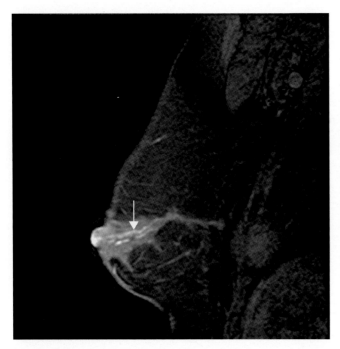

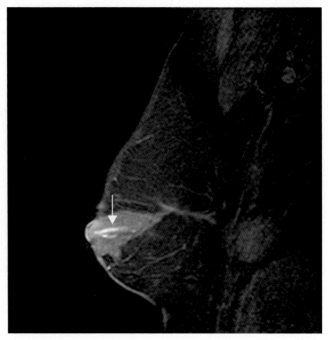

Figure 3.3I   Figure 3.3J

FINDINGS

- Bilateral digital mammogram—a smooth 2-cm mass and with pleiomorphic calcifications is noted in the area of concern. Because these are post-US biopsy images, the clip is within the nodule (Figs. 3.3A–B). US demonstrates a hypoechoic irregular lobulated mass with enhanced through transmission and calcifications (Fig. 3.3C).

WORKUP

- Left breast core biopsy—poorly differentiated invasive duct carcinoma
- Breast MRI for extent of disease evaluation demonstrated the index lesion was a large irregular enhancing mass containing metallic clip with mixed enhancement kinetics including areas of washout (Figs. 3.3G–H). In addition, multiple enhancing nearby nodules highly suspicious for satellite disease were identified with similar enhancing kinetics. The furthest nodule was approximately 3–4 cm posterior to the index lesion (Figs. 3.3E–F).
- She was advised to undergo additional core biopsy of the furthest away suspected lesion before surgery. She opted for lumpectomy and sentinel node biopsy, with wire localization and excisional biopsy of the posterior enhancing focus. Final pathology revealed a 3.0-cm invasive duct adenocarcinoma and an additional 0.2-cm invasive carcinoma from the separate excisional biopsy site, with adequate margins around both sites and 1/13 positive nodes.
- After surgery and final pathology revealed multiple areas of malignancy, she was advised to undergo mastectomy but declined. Oncologic management included radiation therapy.
- She was subsequently followed with annual MRI and 6-month follow-up digital mammography. Two to 3 years later, she developed a new retroareolar area of linear/ductal enhancement that on core biopsy was consistent with DCIS. She subsequently underwent mastectomy for recurrence (Figs. 3.I–J).

DISCUSSION

Doing the extent of disease evaluation can allow for detection of occult lesions that may otherwise not be detected until after the patient has undergone attempted breast conservation. If detected by MRI, such lesions can be addressed before the initial surgery and allow for appropriate planning. When breast carcinoma is multifocal/multicentric, the risk of recurrence after breast cancer treatment is higher. Although this patient initially declined mastectomy, this proved to be necessary 2–3 years later.

• CASE 4

HISTORY

A 71-year-old woman with a family history of a sister with premenopausal breast cancer who presents with a "left breast thickening." Her physical exam is consistent with a palpable asymmetric mass in the 4:00 axis.

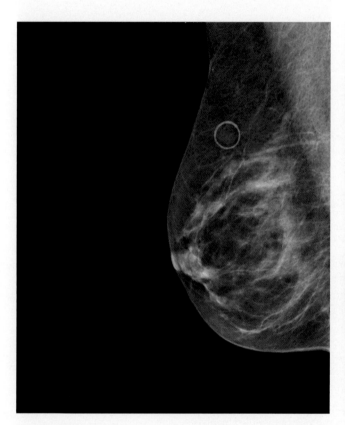

Figure 3.4A

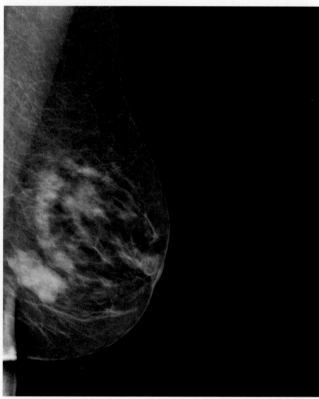

Figure 3.4B

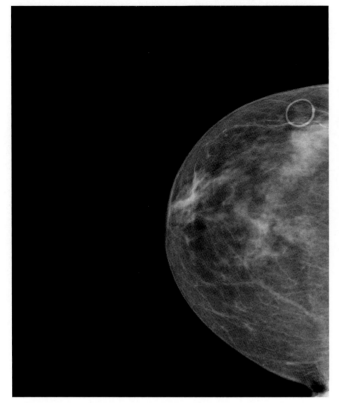

Figure 3.4C

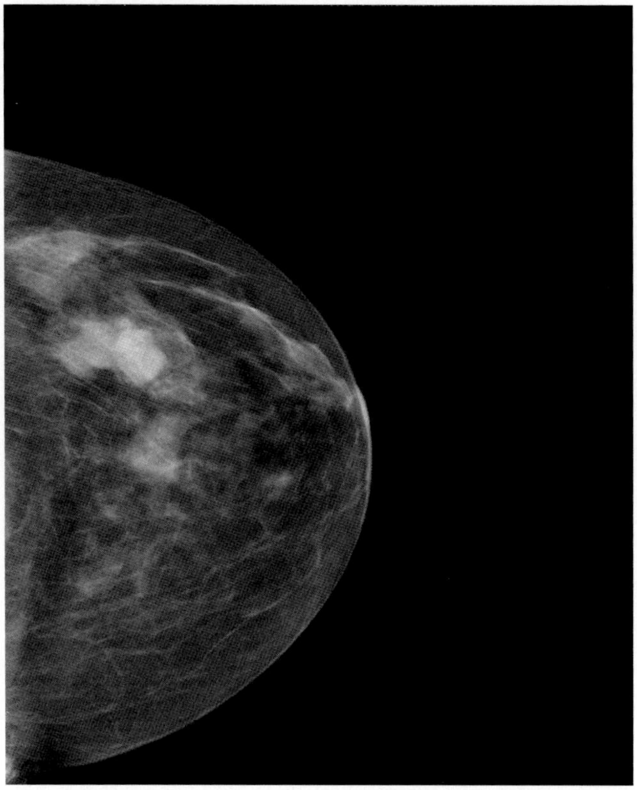

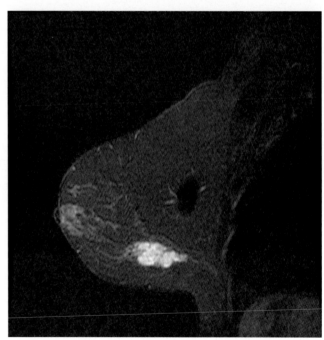

Figure 3.4D

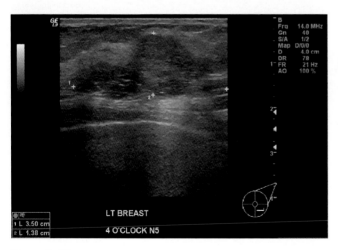

Figure 3.4E

Figure 3.4F

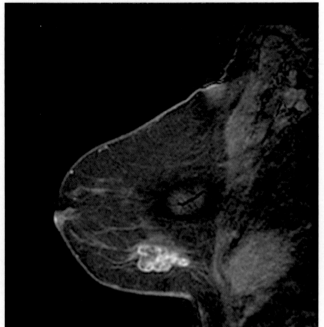

Figure 3.4G

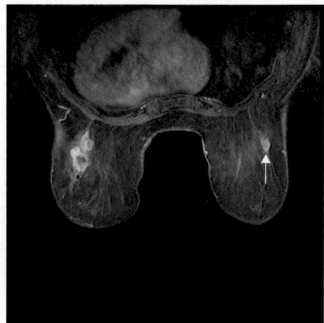

Figure 3.4H

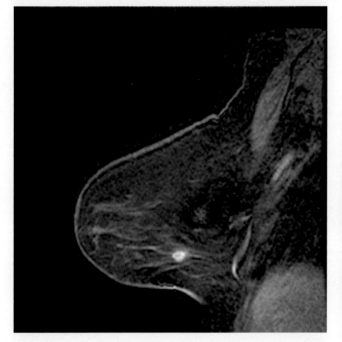

Figure 3.4I

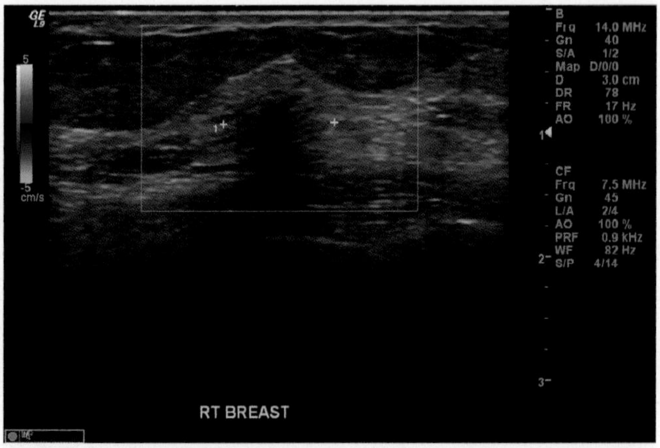

Figure 3.4J

FINDINGS

- Bilateral mammogram (Figs. 3.4A–D)—A 2 × 3 cm macrolobulated mass in the 4:00 position of the left breast with no associated calcifications.
- Left US (Fig. 3.4E)—An irregular mass, hypoechoic, lobulated with areas of increased through transmission, measuring 4.0 cm in maximum diameter.

WORKUP

- Left US core biopsy demonstrated an invasive mucinous carcinoma.
- Breast MRI (Figs. 3.4F–G) for extent of disease evaluation. The MRI demonstrated the index lesion to be a 4-cm macrolobulated-enhancing mass that demonstrated predominantly progressive enhancing kinetics with very high intensity on sagittal STIR (Fig. 3.4F) images. A 1.0-cm, slightly irregular ring-enhancing nodule with washout kinetics was seen in the right outer lower quadrant (Figs. 3.4H–I).
- A targeted right breast US was performed and demonstrated a shadowing lesion that corresponded to the MRI lesion (Fig. 3.4J).
- Right US core biopsy demonstrated invasive ductal carcinoma.
- Patient underwent bilateral lumpectomies with wire localizations and sentinel node biopsies. Final pathology revealed: left, 4.0-cm invasive mucinous/ductal carcinoma with negative sentinel nodes; right, 1.0-cm invasive ductal carcinoma with negative sentinel nodes.

DISCUSSION

Notice the axial images that demonstrate the nearly mirror image location of these two breast cancers. Also, note that the two different pathologies are reflected in the imaging characteristics. The left breast carcinoma demonstrates a high signal on STIR and progressive enhancing kinetics, which are features that are usually associated with benign disease. Mucinous carcinomas are the only malignancy that frequently demonstrates very high signal on STIR (T2). The left breast lesion is not mistaken for a benign lesion however, because of multiple factors including large size, irregular lobulated margin, heterogeneous internal, and ring enhancement. The right breast carcinoma has more typical features of malignancy on MRI, including lower intensity signal on STIR and washout enhancement kinetics.

• CASE 5

HISTORY

A 77-year-old woman with no family history presented with a routine mammogram demonstrating a new right inner posterior mass.

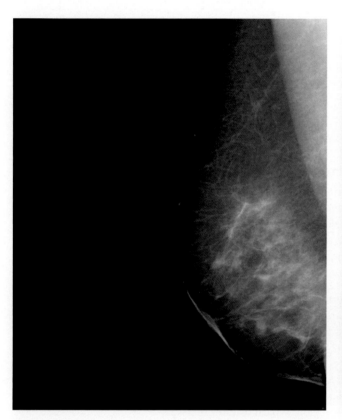

Figure 3.5A

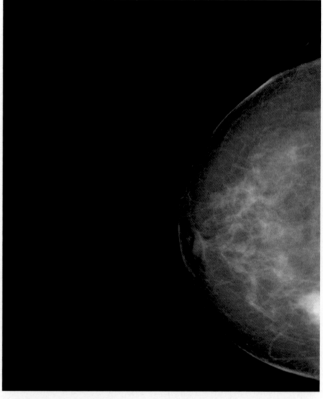

Figure 3.5B

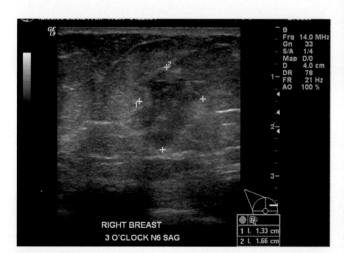
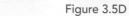

Figure 3.5C

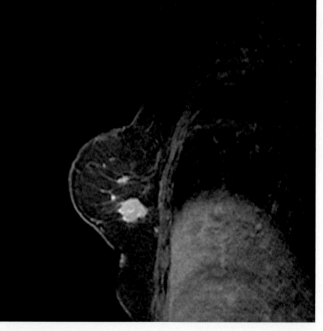

Figure 3.5D

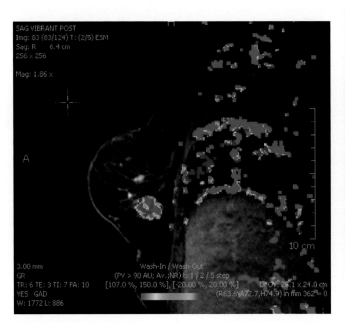

Figure 3.5E

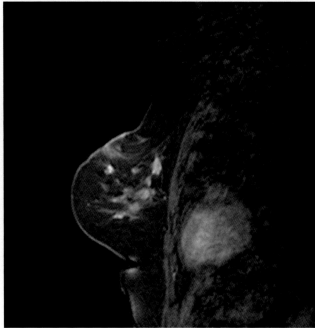

Figure 3.5F

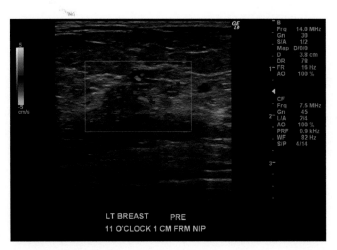

Figure 3.5G

FINDINGS

- Bilateral digital mammography (Figs. 3.5A–B)—The anterior edge of a new rounded right density is seen in the posterior most aspect of the craniocaudal view only, not visualized on the mediolateral view. An inner exaggerated craniocaudal view demonstrates better visualization of this relatively large mass.
- Right US (Fig. 3.5C)—Demonstrates a corresponding hypoechoic mass with slightly thick echogenic rim, and taller than wide configuration.

WORKUP

- Right US-guided core biopsy demonstrated an invasive ductal carcinoma, poorly differentiated.
- MRI—Extent of disease evaluation (Fig. 3.5D): the index lesion is seen in the right inner breast. It is spiculated, heterogeneously enhancing 2.0-cm mass, which demonstrates mostly washout kinetics. There are possible satellite nodules superiorly, enhancing less intensely (Fig. 3.5E). In the opposite breast, there are two to three enhancing nodules (Fig. 3.5F). Targeted left US was performed of this area and demonstrated a hypoechoic shadowing lesion with increased vascularity in the 11:00 axis (Fig. 3.5G).
- US core biopsies were performed and demonstrated multiple sites of invasive carcinoma. She opted for bilateral mastectomies. Final pathology: right (3:00), 3.0 cm invasive ductal carcinoma with DCIS; left (11:00), invasive ductal 0.9 cm, with DCIS, atypical ductal hyperplasia.

DISCUSSION

Even when background enhancement is severe during an extent of disease evaluation, careful search needs to be made for additional/contralateral lesions. Because delaying scan for ideal phase of menstrual cycle not feasible for extent of disease scans (because of timing for surgery), background enhancement can be more problematic. In these cases, the kinetics may help distinguish an area of nodular breast tissues from a suspicious area. Use margin analysis (checking for spiculations or irregularity) in both the axial and sagittal series.

• CASE 6

HISTORY

An 82-year-old woman with no prior mammographic screens presents with intense, focal right breast pain.

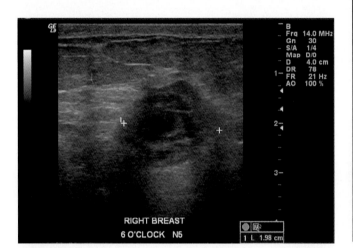

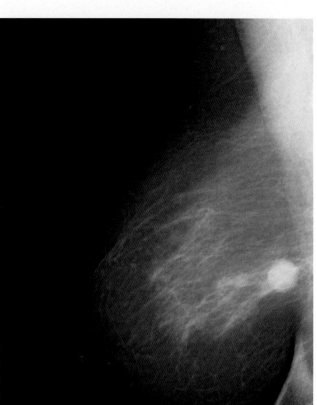

Figure 3.6A

Figure 3.6B

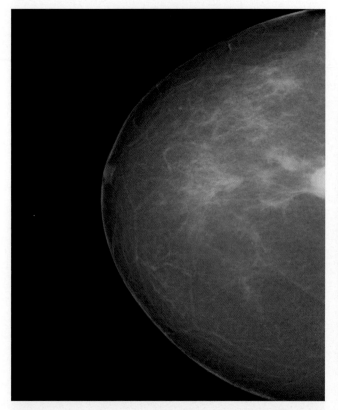

Figure 3.6C

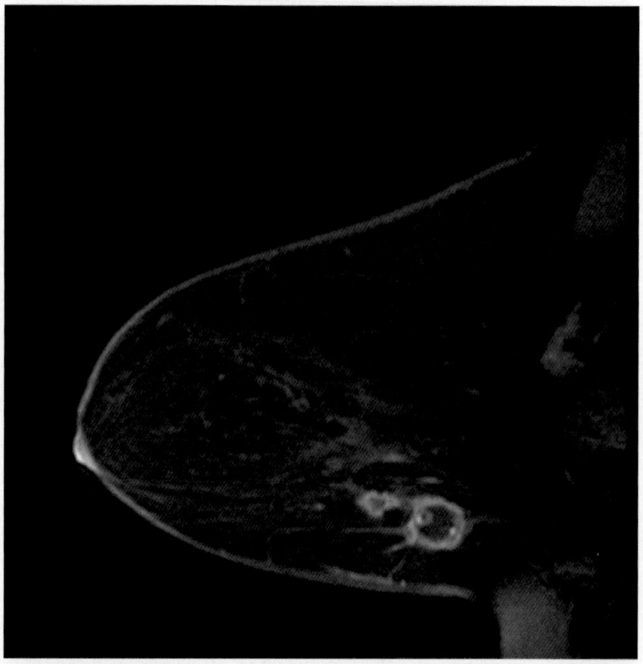

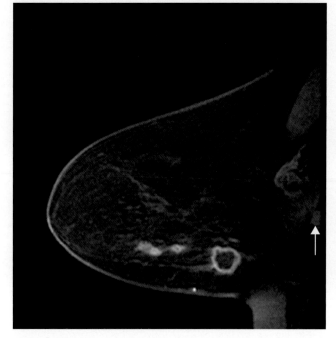

Figure 3.6E

Figure 3.6D

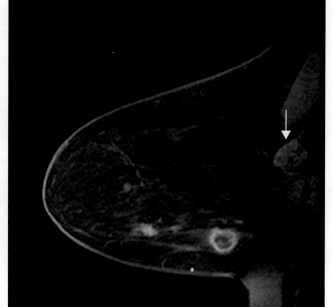

Figure 3.6F

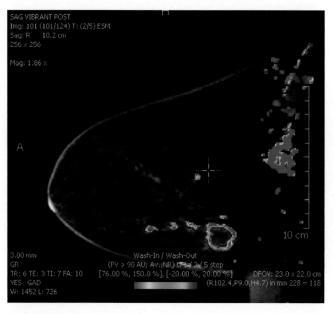
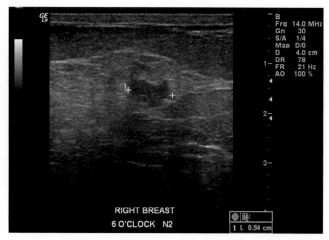

Figure 3.6G

FINDINGS

- Bilateral US—Demonstrated a large thick-walled mass (right breast 6:00 axis) with necrotic center, highly suspicious for malignancy (Fig. 3.6A).
- Bilateral digital mammography—Demonstrated fatty breasts with a dominant mass in the posterior third of the right lower breast and nodular asymmetric tissue with additional smaller nodular densities extending anteriorly (Figs. 3.6B–C).

WORKUP

- US-guided core biopsy was performed demonstrating an invasive ductal carcinoma.
- MRI—Demonstrated in addition to the large ring-enhancing mass compatible with recently diagnosed carcinoma (Figs. 3.06D–F) approximately six additional suspicious enhancing nodules, the largest of which has ring enhancement. All were in a segmental distribution. In addition, marked axillary adenopathy and even mediastinal adenopathy is noted.
- Color kinetics demonstrate very heterogeneous kinetics, with areas of washout. Notice the satellite lesions display a very similar pattern of enhancement kinetics (Fig. 3.6G).
- She underwent mastectomy—Final pathology revealed multicentric invasive carcinoma, with extensive axillary involvement.

DISCUSSION

Even though the focus of breast MRI is extent of disease in the breasts, check other areas for disease such as axilla, ribs, and mediastinum. If there is evidence of axillary adenopathy, try to document metastatic disease before surgery to avoid an unnecessary sentinel node biopsy. If axillary mets are suspected, perform a targeted US of axilla. Any lymph node that demonstrates a thickened cortex should be considered suspicious and evaluated with needle biopsy. If possible bone lesions are present, evaluate with nuclear bone scan. Suspected mediastinal or pulmonary lesions can be evaluated with chest computed tomography. Fine-needle aspiration biopsy is sufficient for axillary metastasis from invasive ductal carcinoma; for invasive lobular CA, cytology is less precise, so consider performing a small-gauge core biopsy if it can be done safely. (Even though patients can be reluctant to undergo multiple needle biopsies, they are more reluctant to have multiple surgical procedures.) As much of the workup as possible should be done in radiology department, before the surgical procedure; you may help the surgeon avoid subjecting the patient to multiple trips to the operating room.

• CASE 7

HISTORY

A 70-year-old woman who presented with clustered calcifications on screening mammogram. Stereotactic biopsy demonstrated invasive ductal carcinoma.

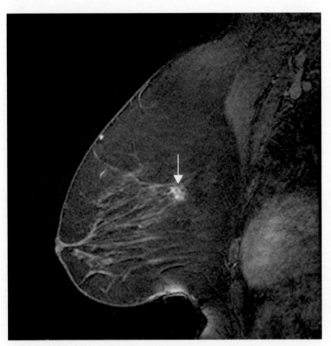

Figure 3.7A

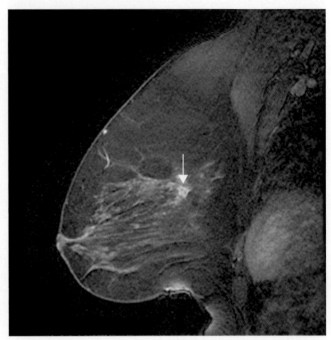

Figure 3.7B

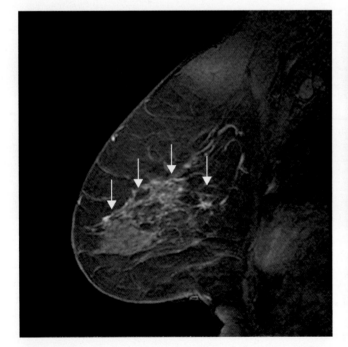

Figure 3.7C

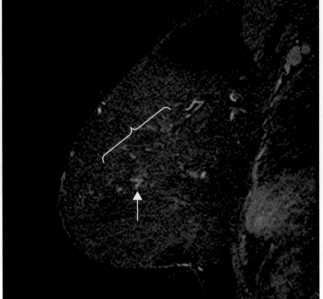

Figure 3.7D

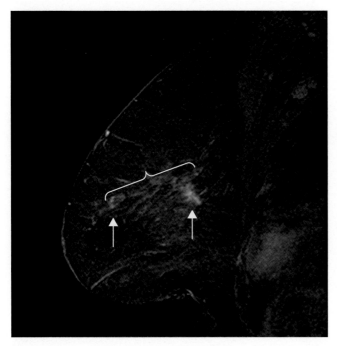

Figure 3.7E

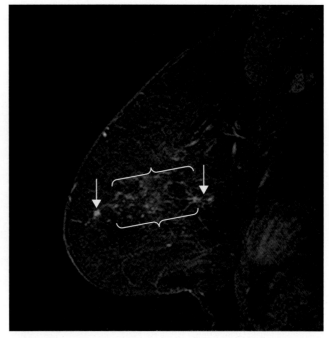

Figure 3.7F

FINDINGS

- MRI—Demonstrated a 1-cm highly spiculated irregular enhancing lesion (Figs. 3.7A–B) corresponding to the clinically known carcinoma. In addition, there is a large region of subtle grouped ("clustered") progressively enhancing foci in a segmental distribution throughout the upper half of the breast (Figs. 3.7C–F). This is more conspicuous on subtraction images. Be suspicious of surrounding DCIS (Figs. 3.7C–F) whenever this appearance is noted. We call this the "dot-dash pattern" appearance of DCIS. The patient declined additional core biopsies and instead wanted attempted lumpectomy. After multiple attempts at obtaining clear margins for extensive DCIS, she underwent mastectomy.

DISCUSSION

The appearance of DCIS surrounding a known carcinoma can be very subtle. Be sure to check the last postcontrast series as the enhancement of the surrounding DCIS may be much slower and therefore more evident later on. Occasionally, areas of DCIS without invasion can appear to be masslike and spiculated on MRI.

• Plate 1

HISTORY

A 54-year-old woman, asymptomatic, presented with abnormalities on routine imaging.

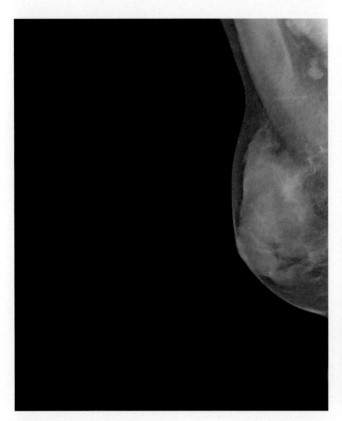

Plate 3.1A

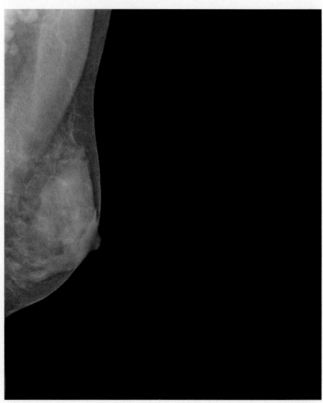

Plate 3.1B

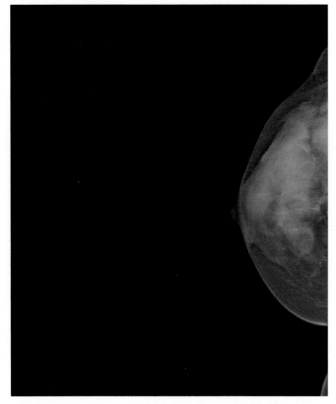

Plate 3.1C

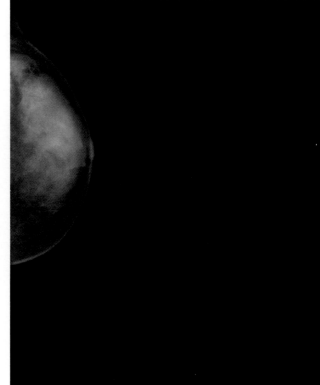

Plate 3.1D

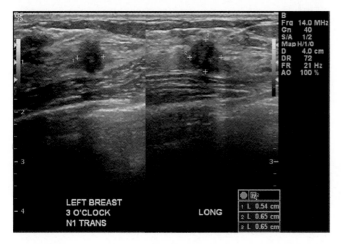

Plate 3.1E

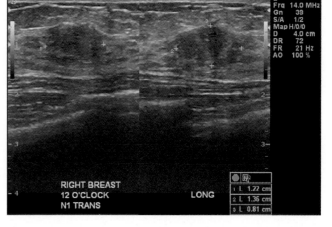

Plate 3.1F

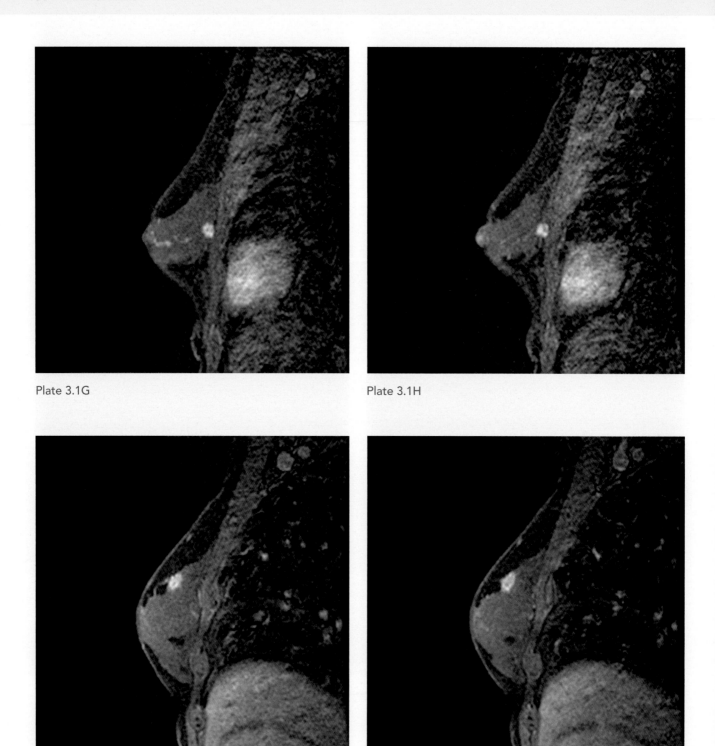

Plate 3.1G

Plate 3.1H

Plate 3.1I

Plate 3.1J

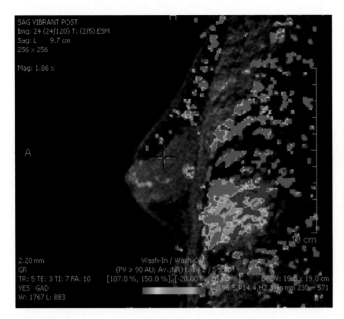

Plate 3.1K

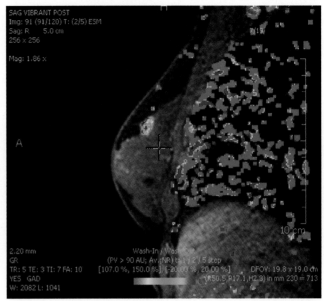

Plate 3.1L

FINDINGS

- Plates 3.1A–D—Bilateral digital mammography demonstrated dense breasts, but was otherwise negative and unchanged from prior exams. US screening was suggested because of extremely dense breast parenchyma.

- Plate 3.1E—Selected images from bilateral screening US demonstrated a suspicious irregular 7-mm hypoechoic shadowing left mass and an ovoid indeterminant right mass.

- Bilateral US core biopsy was performed.

- Plates 3.1G–J—Selected images from bilateral breast MRI done as extent of disease evaluation demonstrates highly suspicious irregular bilateral enhancing masses, with spiculated margins and very heterogeneous enhancement kinetics, consistent with bilateral carcinoma (Plates 3.01K–L).

- Notice that the masses both demonstrate predominately plateau enhancement kinetics, but the left contains more areas of washout than the right.

FINAL PATHOLOGY

- Right breast core biopsy—Invasive ductal carcinoma, ER 94%+, PR 10%+, HER-2/neu 1+, Ki-67 22%.

- Left breast core biopsy—Invasive ductal carcinoma, ER 97%+, PR 58%+, HER-2/neu 2+, Ki-67 22%.

• Plate 2

HISTORY

A 48-year-old asymptomatic woman with a family history for breast cancer presents for routine imaging.

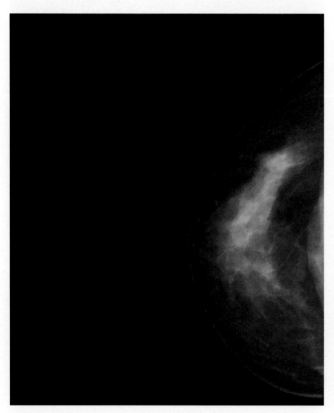

Plate 3.2A

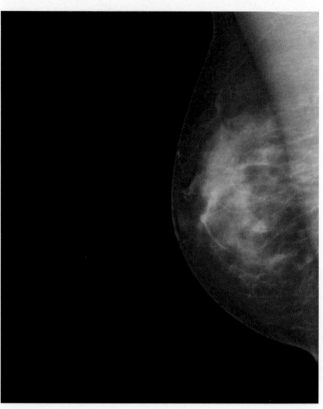

Plate 3.2B

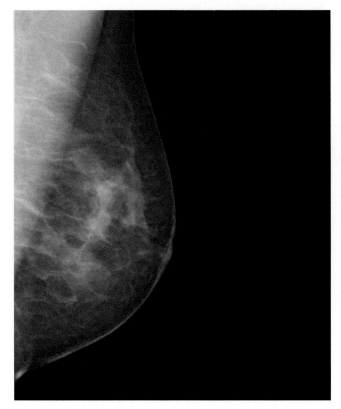

Plate 3.2C

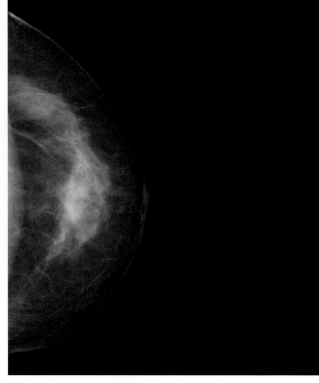

Plate 3.2D

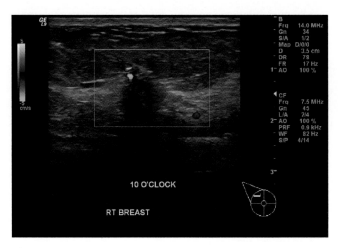

Plate 3.2E

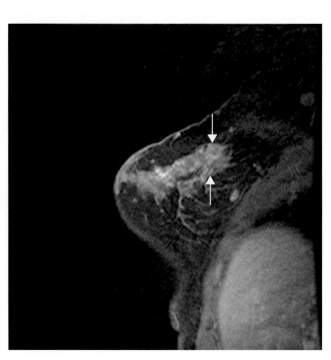

Plate 3.2F

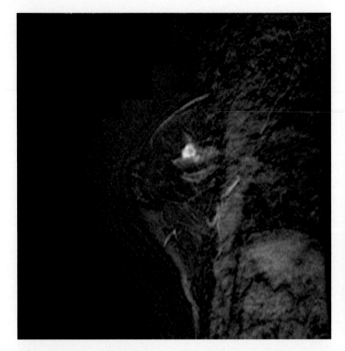

Plate 3.2G

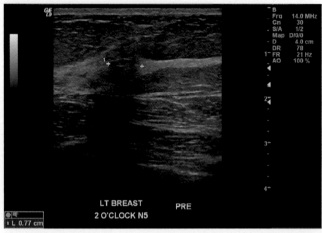

Plate 3.2H

FINDINGS

- Plates 3.2A–D—Mammogram: heterogeneously dense breasts, negative.
- Plate 3.2E—Screening breast US demonstrated a highly suspicious, poorly defined, irregular shadowing lesion with increased vascularity in the right upper outer quadrant. US core biopsy consistent with invasive lobular carcinoma.
- Plate 3.2F—MRI of the right breast demonstrating the index lesion: faintly progressive grouped or clustered enhancing linear and nodular foci. Lobular carcinomas may enhance minimally as seen in this case.
- Plate 3.2G—Left MRI demonstrates a ring-enhancing irregular 1.1-cm left upper outer quadrant mass with washout kinetics, highly suspicious for contralateral synchronous carcinoma.
- Plate 3.2H—Left breast-targeted US demonstrated a hypoechoic shadowing area that corresponded to MRI lesion. US core biopsy demonstrated invasive ductal carcinoma.

FINAL PATHOLOGY

- Right—1.2-cm invasive lobular, lobular carcinoma in situ, and one positive sentinel node.
- Left—0.9-cm invasive ductal, no positive nodes.

COMMENTS

- If a patient presents with newly diagnosed carcinoma, there is a 3–5% chance of an occult synchronous contralateral carcinoma.
- Lobular carcinomas occasionally are non-enhancing, and may result in a false negative MRI.

• Plate 3

HISTORY

A 70-year-old woman who presented with a palpable abnormality in the right lower outer breast approximately 6 months after negative recent mammographic screen.

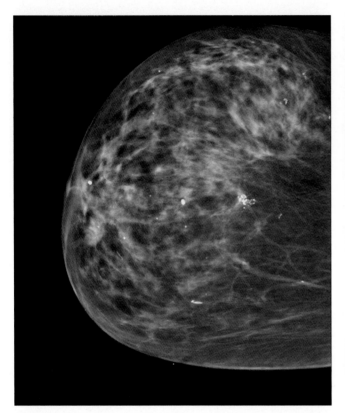

Plate 3.3A

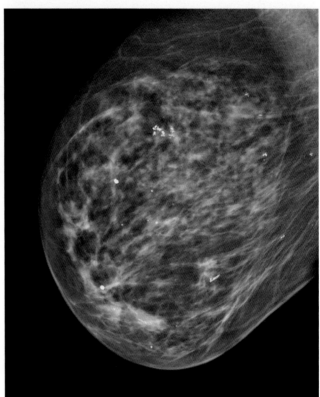

Plate 3.3B

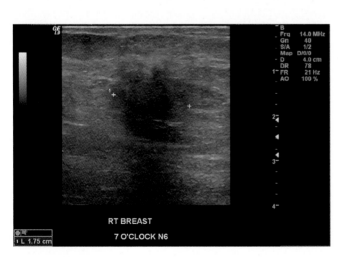

Plate 3.3C

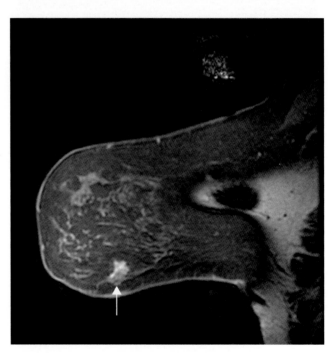

Plate 3.3D

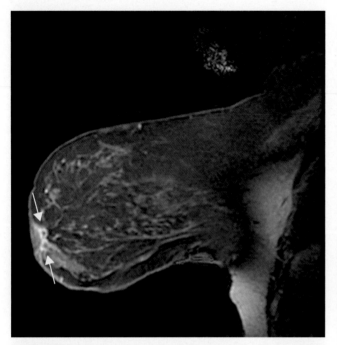

Plate 3.3E

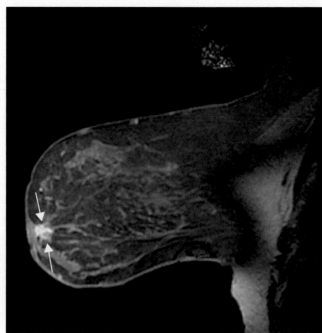

Plate 3.3F

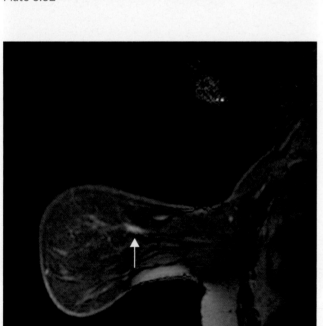

Plate 3.3G

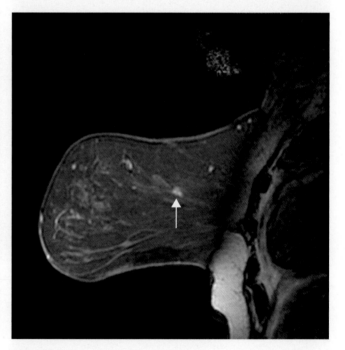

Plate 3.3H

FINDINGS

- Plates 3.3A–B—Digital mammogram showed heterogeneously dense nodular breasts without suspicious findings or interval change from prior exams.

- Plate 3.3C—Right US demonstrated a shadowing area with increase vascularity that corresponded to the palpable mass; subsequent core biopsy of this area demonstrated an invasive lobular carcinoma.

- Plate 3.3D—Postcontrast sagittal image demonstrates a spiculated enhancing mass in the right outer lower quadrant corresponding to the recently biopsied carcinoma.

- Plates 3.3E–F—In the right breast, a second enhancing retroareolar mass is seen with irregular spiculated margins, heterogeneous internal enhancement, and possible nipple retraction. Target US and US core demonstrated a second area of invasive lobular carcinoma.

- Plate 3.3G—A third lesion is demonstrated as an irregular area of linear enhancement in the right (inner upper quadrant) breast. This linear pattern suggests a ductal configuration. This can be differentiated from a vessel in that the linear enhancement is thicker and has a beaded or irregular appearance. Also, it cannot be traced anteriorly and posteriorly as a vessel would on consecutive sections. Targeted US and US core demonstrated DCIS.

- Plate 3.3H—A fourth lesion is seen as a small enhancing nodule in the opposite breast. Even a lesion that may not appear to be obviously malignant should be viewed with a suspicion in the setting of extent of disease evaluation. This lesion proved to be an invasive ductal carcinoma.

DISCUSSION

In a case such as this with multiple suspicious lesions, we biopsy the most suspicious synchronous lesion (or lesions) first. If this is positive, then biopsy the second most suspicious area, and so on. After multicentric (multiquadrant disease) is established, however, no further sampling is necessary because mastectomy becomes the treatment of choice. When using MRI for extent of disease, consider the overall surgical plan as well as the individual patient.

• Plate 4

HISTORY

A 55-year-old woman with bilateral scarring in breast from prior burns and surgical treatments from a foreign country.

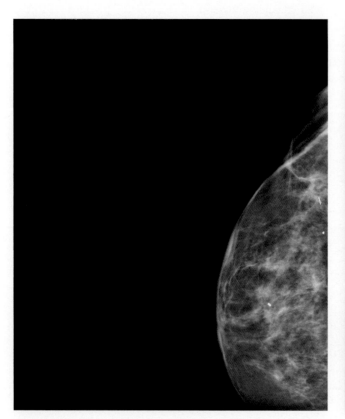

Plate 3.4A

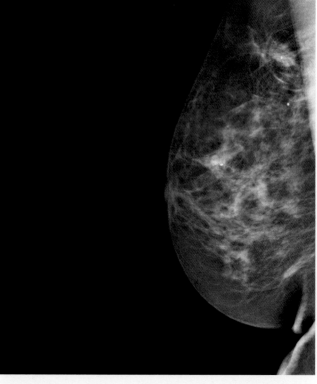

Plate 3.4B

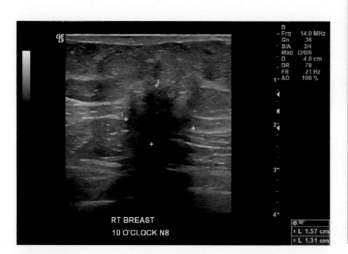

Plate 3.4C

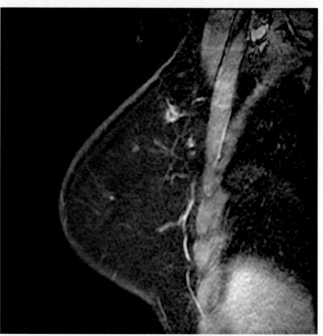

Plate 3.4D

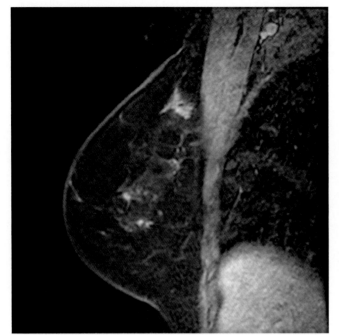

Plate 3.4E

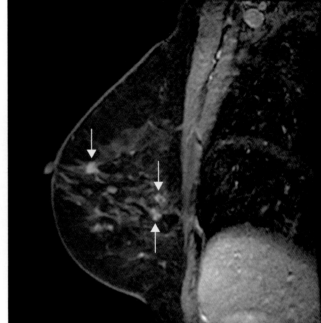

Plate 3.4F

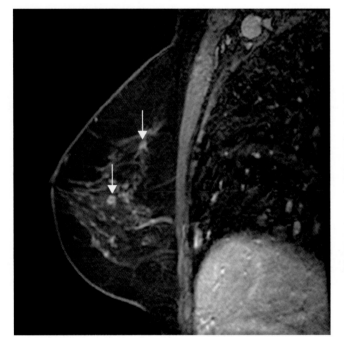

Plate 3.4G

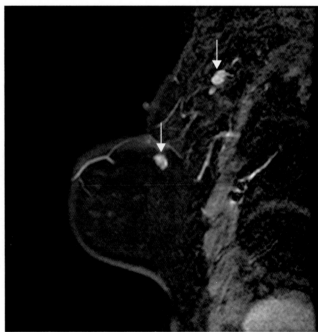

Plate 3.4H

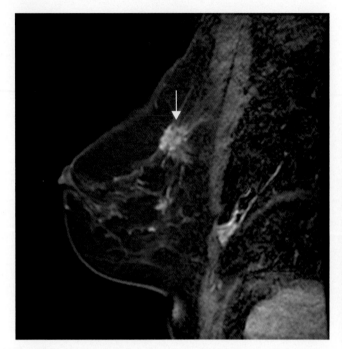

Plate 3.4I

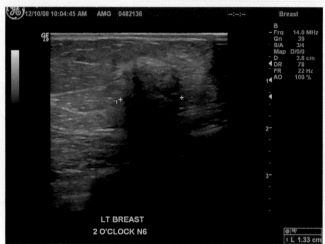

Plate 3.4J

FINDINGS

- Plates 3.4A–B—Right mammogram: areas thought previously to correspond to scarring appeared more prominent than on prior exams. These are images after US-guided biopsies were performed, so clips are present.

- Plate 3.4C—US demonstrating an irregular hypoechoic shadowing lesion in the area thought to be scar on mammogram. Core biopsy was consistent with invasive ductal carcinoma.

- Plates 3.4D–I—Breast MRI depicted demonstrated numerous bilateral lesions. Targeted US was performed and multiple US-guided biopsies were performed.

- Plate 3.4J—Shadowing mass is noted in the left upper outer quadrant. Multiple other bilateral nodules were sampled using US guidance; all were positive for malignancy.

DISCUSSION

Patient underwent bilateral mastectomies. Final pathology demonstrated multifocal invasive ductal carcinoma on the right and three masses consistent with invasive ductal (two) and invasive lobular (one) carcinomas on the left.

• CASE 1

HISTORY

A 54-year-old woman with no family history of breast cancer who presents after a bilateral breast reduction. Her pathology revealed an incidental finding of two foci of ductal carcinoma in situ (DCIS), intermediate to high nuclear grade, right breast. No other localizing information (e.g., quadrant) was available from pathology. She has a history of hormone replacement therapy for 11 years.

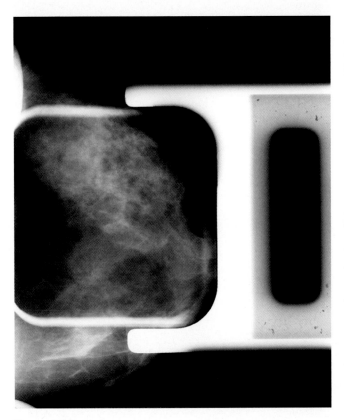

Figure 4.1A

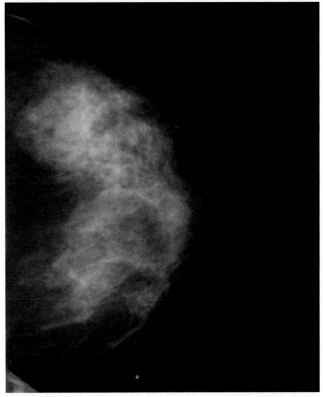

Figure 4.1B

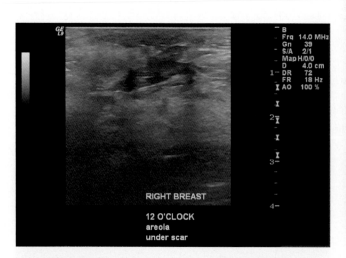

Figure 4.1C

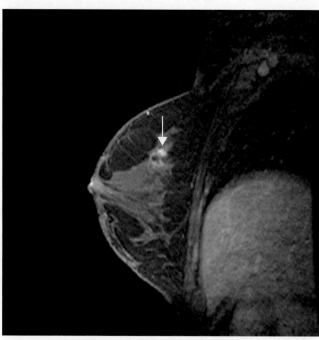

Figure 4.1D

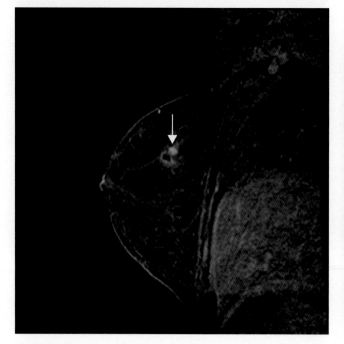

Figure 4.1E

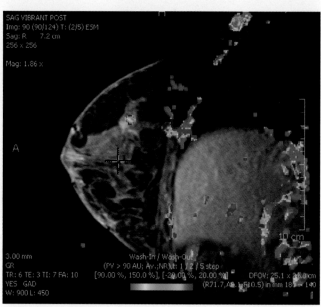

Figure 4.1F

FINDINGS

- Mammogram—Negative before reduction. On postreduction, demonstrated dense breasts with postsurgical changes (Figs. 4.1A–B).

- Breast ultrasound (US) demonstrated only postsurgical changes (Fig. 4.1C).

- Breast MRI—Demonstrated a 6-mm nodule in the right upper breast with very heterogeneous enhancement kinetics (Figs. 4.1D–F).

WORKUP

- Patient underwent a magnetic resonance image (MRI)-guided wire localization with excisional biopsy which demonstrated 6-mm well-differentiated invasive ductal carcinoma with a separate focus of a 4-mm DCIS.

- She opted for breast conservation and sentinel node biopsy.

DISCUSSION

After extensive surgery, mammogram and US have very limited role in evaluation for breast abnormality, because postsurgical changes obscure visualization. One of the initial uses of MRI was to distinguish scar from recurrent disease, and MRI is still the most useful tool in evaluating postoperative breasts. In this case, despite rim-enhancing postsurgical collections and areas of low-grade, less-intense postsurgical enhancement, a discrete intensely enhancing 6-mm nodule is readily visible. Without MRI, it may take 1 to 2 years or longer for this carcinoma to be apparent on mammographic/clinical/sonographic exam.

• CASE 2

HISTORY

A 45-year-old woman presents with a questionable distortion on screening mammogram. She denies a family history or personal history of breast cancer.

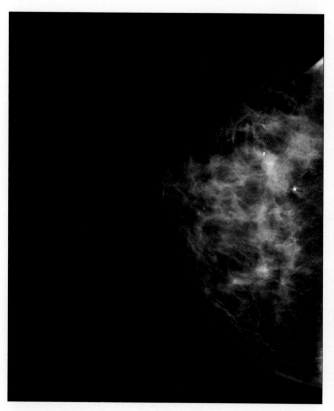

Figure 4.2A

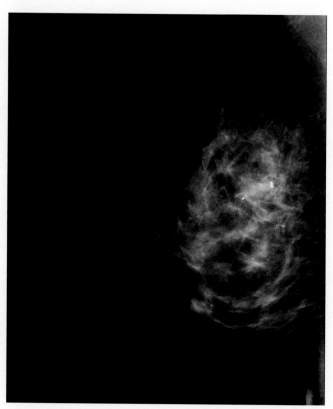

Figure 4.2B

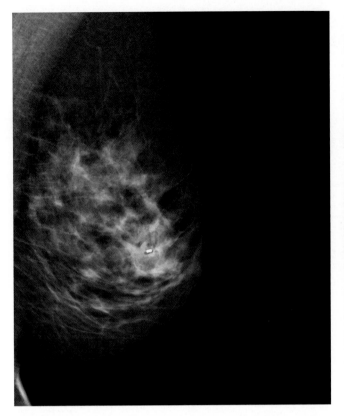

Figure 4.2C

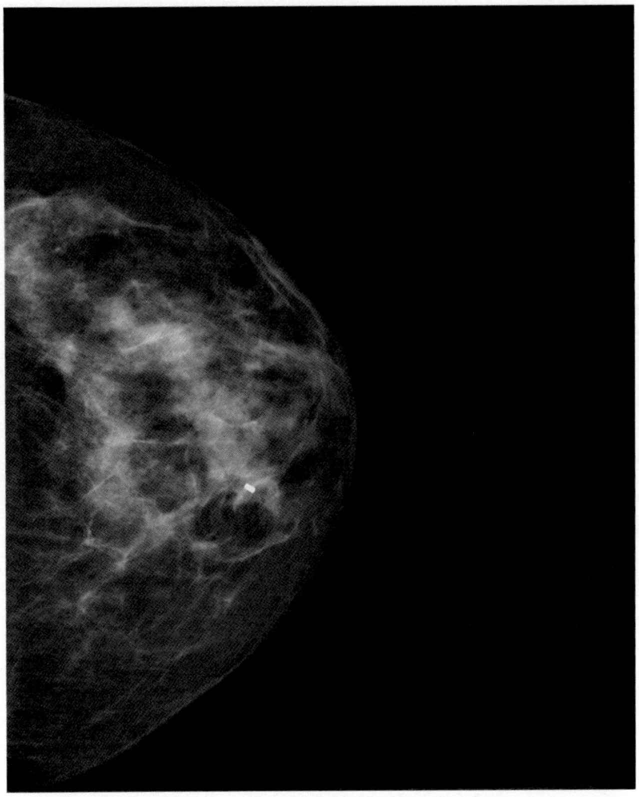

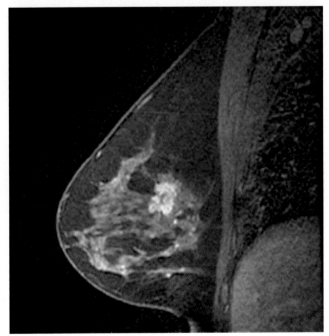

Figure 4.2D

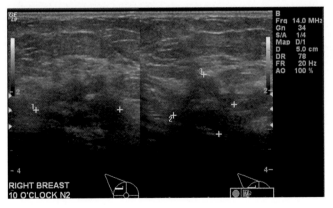

Figure 4.2E

Figure 4.2F

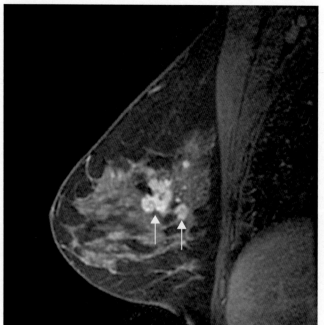

Figure 4.2G

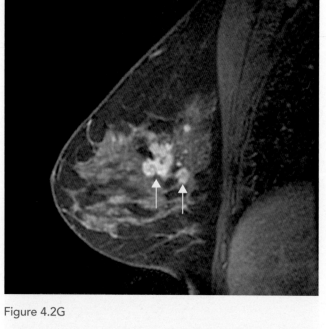

Figure 4.2H

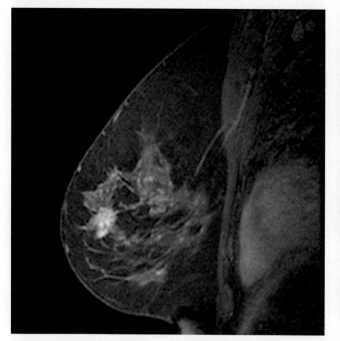

Figure 4.2I

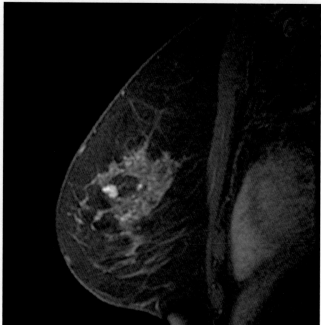

Figure 4.2J

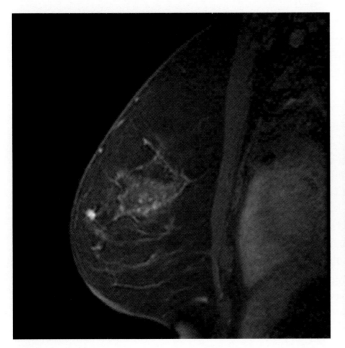

Figure 4.2K

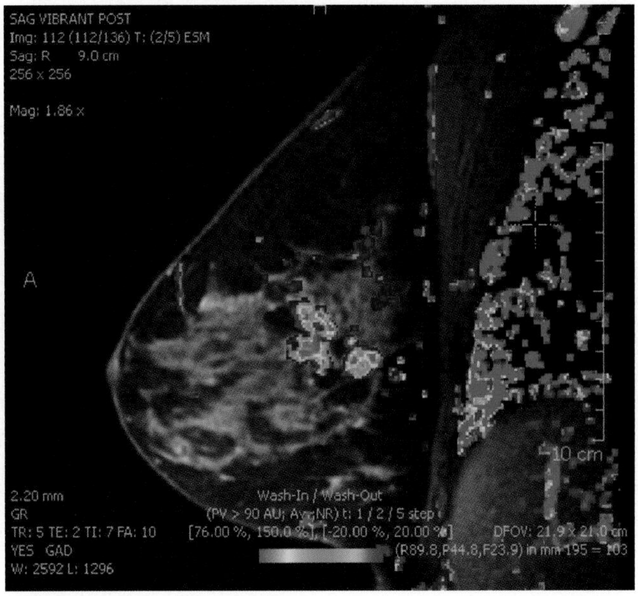

Figure 4.2L

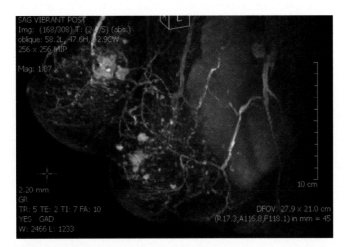

Figure 4.2M

FINDINGS

- Right mammogram—Demonstrated architectural distortion (Figs. 4.2A–B). Left mammogram was negative (Figs. 4.2C–D). Postbiopsy images are displayed, so that the reader can appreciate the sites that were later seen to correspond to enhancing areas and biopsied.

- Right US —A vague hypoechoic shadowing region measuring approximately 2 cm is seen (Fig. 4.2E). (She had a right US-guided core biopsy that was benign but discordant.)

- Breast MRI—Performed as a problem-solving exam for discordant result from ultrasound guided biopsy, and demonstrated two spiculated masses in the right outer upper quadrant, in the area of concern (Figs. 4.2F–H). Also seen are possible smaller satellite lesions (superiorly). In addition, there were three highly suspicious enhancing masses in the left inner breast (Figs. 4.2I–K).

- Figure 4.2L—Color enhanced computer aided diagnosis image demonstrates markedly heterogeneous enhancement kinetics including areas of washout.

- Figure 4.2M—Demonstrates three-dimensional computer aided diagnosis image depicting multiple bilateral masses. This allows clinicians (and patients when appropriate) to truly appreciate the extent of disease.

WORKUP

- Patient underwent MRI-guided core biopsies of the left and right abnormalities.

- Final pathology revealed bilateral multifocal invasive ductal carcinoma, moderately differentiated.

- She opted for bilateral mastectomies. Final pathology demonstrated three areas of invasive ductal carcinoma on the right—1.7, 1.0 and 0.5 cm—and on the left, an infiltrating moderately differentiated ductal carcinoma in four separate areas, measuring 1.7, 0.3, 0.2, and 1.5 cm.

DISCUSSION

US-guided biopsy was hampered by extreme posterior location and vague borders of the hypoechoic region.

When recommending an excisional biopsy for a discordant lesion, consider obtaining MRI before surgery, for multiple reasons. First, the diagnosis may become more obvious on MRI, as seen in this case. On MRI, the area is clearly consistent with a large right breast carcinoma with satellite lesions. Second, other abnormalities that may require surgical intervention can be revealed preoperatively and addressed during the same surgical procedure. (As in this case, multiple bilateral lesions were detected and worked up before definitive surgery.) Finally, a lesion that may be difficult to target with needle biopsy on digital mammography or US, may be obvious and more easily targeted for core biopsy on MRI. In this case, MRI helped avoid multiple surgeries in this woman with multicentric bilateral breast carcinoma.

• CASE 3

HISTORY

A 79-year-old woman who presents with a history of left bloody nipple discharge intermittently for 3 months.

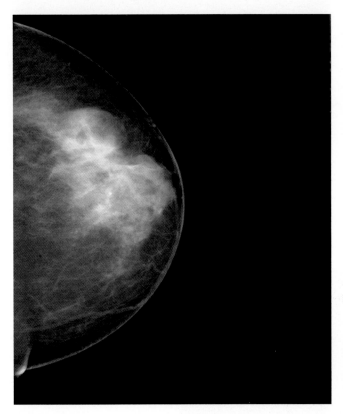

Figure 4.3A

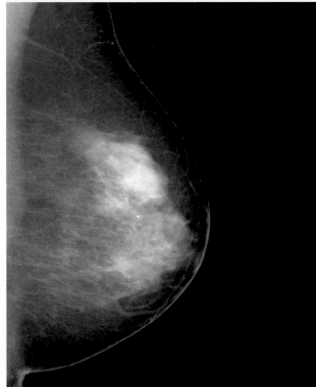

Figure 4.3B

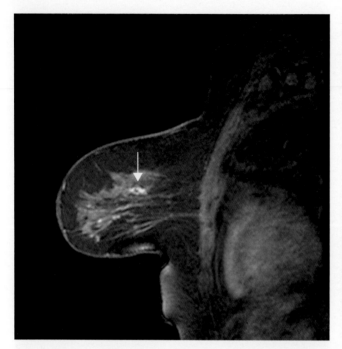

Figure 4.3C

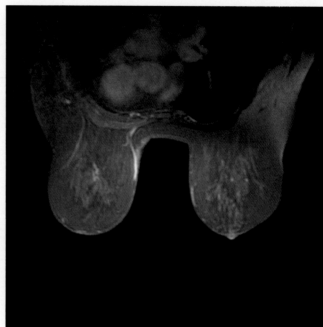

Figure 4.3D

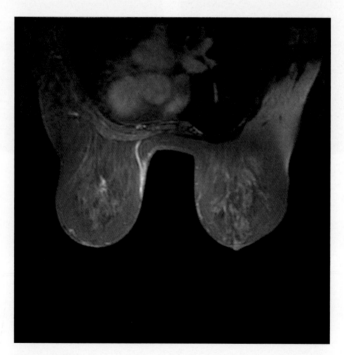

Figure 4.3E

FINDINGS

- Bilateral mammogram—Recent screening (6 months prior) was negative. These images are obtained after attempted US core biopsy (Figs. 4.3A–B).

- She underwent a diagnostic left mammogram and US that demonstrated dense breasts on mammogram and minimal retroareolar ductal ectasia on ultrasound, but no suspicious findings.

- Breast MRI—Demonstrated a 9 × 4-mm area of progressive clumped enhancement with irregular margin in the left upper breast for which core biopsy was recommended (Figs. 4.3C–E). There were no other abnormal areas noted.

WORKUP

- Patient subsequently underwent targeted US, and US-guided core biopsy was performed. However, postbiopsy images revealed the location of the clip did not correspond to the enhancing lesion on MRI.

- She then underwent a MRI-guided needle localization and excision for the abnormal area on MRI, along with a left terminal duct excision for the bloody nipple discharge.

- The MRI lesion was consistent with a 5-mm invasive ductal carcinoma. The terminal duct specimen contained an intraductal papilloma.

- She opted for breast conservation and sentinel node biopsy.

DISCUSSION

Targeted US for small- to medium-sized MRI abnormalities may demonstrate potential corresponding hypoechoic areas that eventually are seen to *not* coincide with the MRI abnormality. When a patient has already undergone one negative needle biopsy, she is often reluctant to undergo a second attempt. Therefore, we now rarely perform targeted US for lesions smaller than 1 cm. Even in larger lesions, the target is often so much more conspicuous on MRI that it significantly improves the accuracy of the biopsy. In the absence of cost concerns, a benign biopsy result from a targeted US finding should ideally be followed by a postbiopsy MRI to confirm the clip is within the enhancing lesion. The marked changes in the configuration of the breast between prone imaging during MRI and supine imaging in US make it hazardous to assume that small lesions found on targeted US in fact correspond to the MRI finding.

Clinically significant nipple discharge with no mammographic or US abnormality should be evaluated with MRI before surgical intervention (terminal duct excision).

• CASE 4

HISTORY

An 81-year-old woman presents with a history of intermittent breast pain for which bilateral mammogram and US was found to be negative. During a workup for chest discomfort, chest computed tomography (CT) was performed that demonstrated a right upper lobe nodule. A positron emission tomography (PET) scan was then performed that demonstrated an area of increased activity in the left breast.

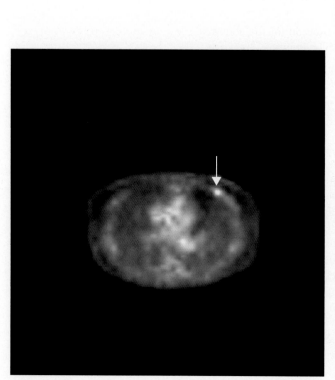

Figure 4.4A

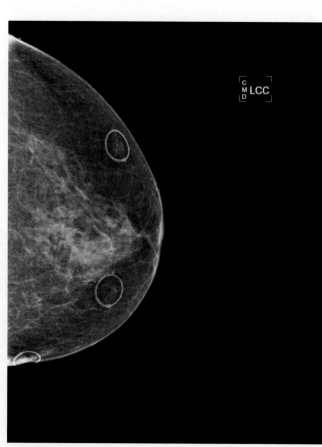

Figure 4.4B

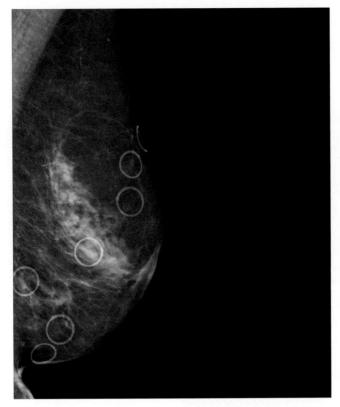

Figure 4.4C

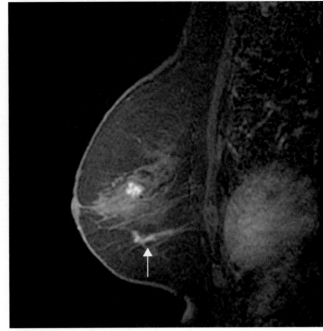

Figure 4.4D

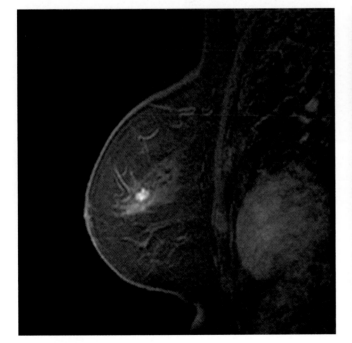

Figure 4.4E

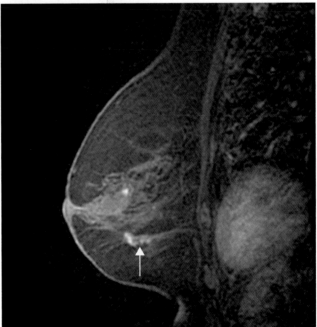

Figure 4.4F

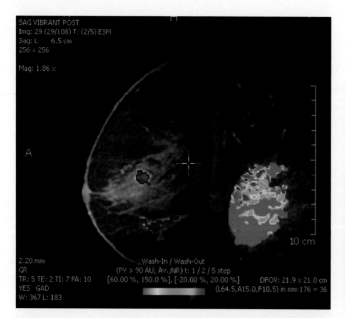

Figure 4.4G

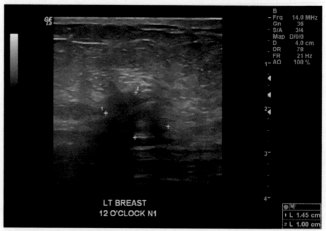

Figure 4.4H

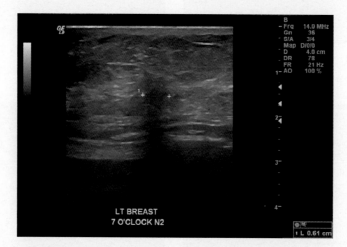

Figure 4.4I

FINDINGS

- PET CT (Fig. 4.4A)—Focal increased activity left breast.

- Mammogram (Figs. 4.4B–C)—Demonstrated breasts composed of mixed fibroglandular and fatty tissue without any suspicious findings or interval changes.

- Breast MRI—Demonstrated two irregular enhancing lesions in the left central breast, with a 1.5-cm enhancing mass along the 12:00 axis and an area of linear and clumped enhancement along the approximately 6:00 axis. Predominantly progressive enhancement kinetics were noted in the superior lesion as well as the 6:00 lesion (Figs. 4.4D–F).

- Targeted US revealed a hypoechoic shadowing, 1.5-cm, poorly defined region in the 12:00 axis, and a smaller shadowing irregular lesion in the 6:00–7:00 axis (Figs. 4.5H–I).

WORKUP

- Core biopsy was performed on both and demonstrated histologically different carcinomas: the 12:00 was invasive poorly differentiated carcinoma; the 6:00 to 7:00, moderately differentiated carcinoma.

- Her definitive surgery was a left total mastectomy that demonstrated, on final pathology, histologically differing invasive carcinomia a 1.4-cm lesion at 12:00 and a 1.2-cm lesion at 6:00 with associated DCIS.

DISCUSSION

- Although the breast density on digital mammography was relatively low, this fairly large mass that is readily visible on MRI was *not* apparent on mammogram.

- The absence of suspicious enhancement kinetics should not dissuade one from performing appropriate follow-up (biopsy) of morphologically suspicious lesions.

- If a significantly suspicious finding is revealed on any imaging modality (e.g., CT scan, PET) that cannot be definitively explained on digital mammography or sonography, MRI scan should be obtained to complete the evaluation and rule out carcinoma.

• **CASE 5**

HISTORY

A 71-year-old woman who has a family history of sister with postmenopausal breast cancer, and two maternal cousins with postmenopausal breast cancer. She had not been undergoing high-risk screening with breast MRI.

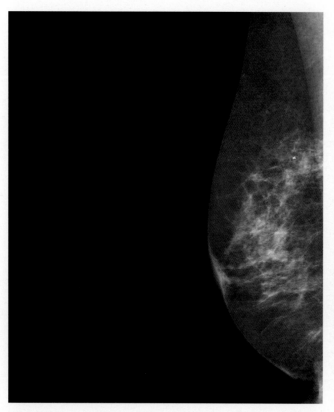

Figure 4.5A

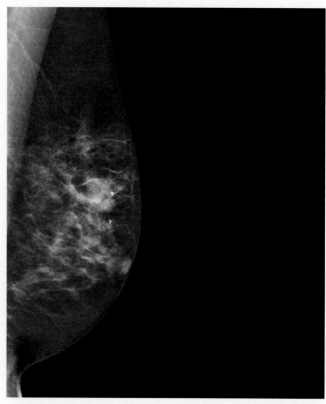

Figure 4.5B

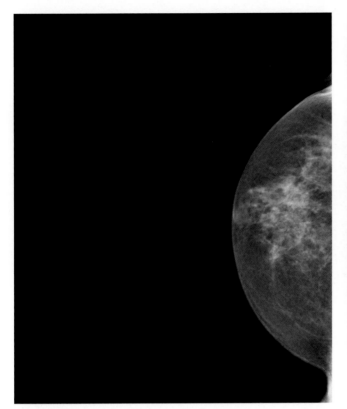

Figure 4.5C

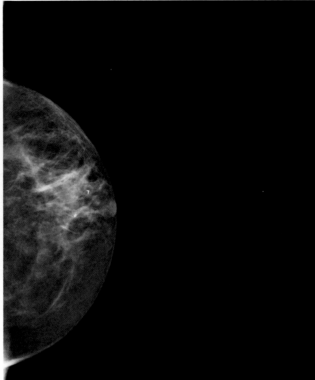

Figure 4.5D

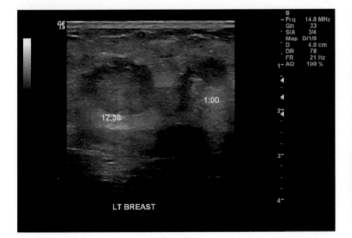

Figure 4.5E

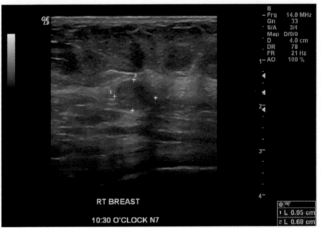

Figure 4.5F

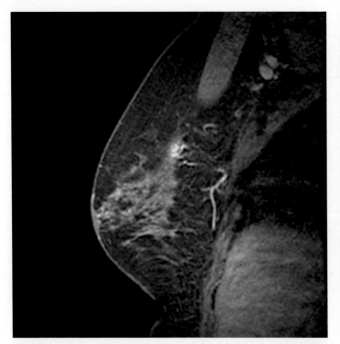

Figure 4.5G

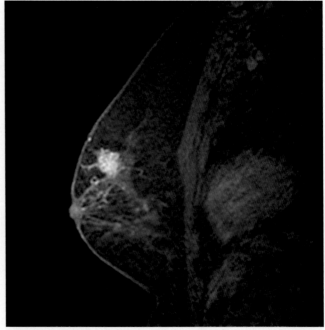

Figure 4.5H

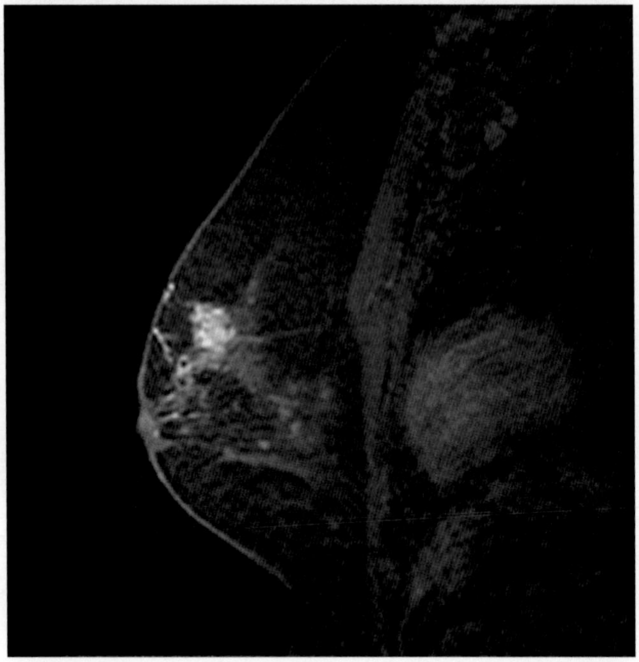

Figure 4.5I

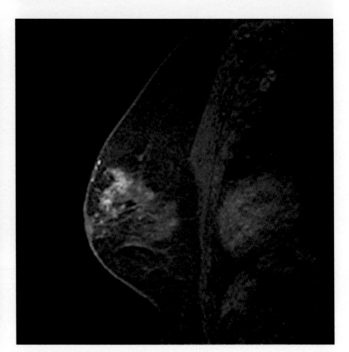

Figure 4.5J

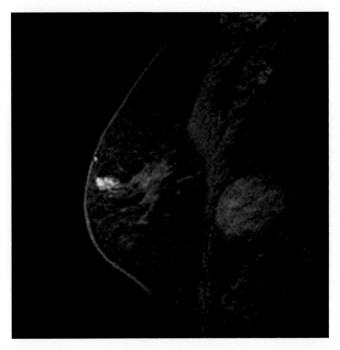

Figure 4.5K

FINDINGS

- Bilateral mammogram demonstrated asymmetric nodular areas bilaterally: left, upper outer; right, upper breast (Figs. 4.5A–D).
- Bilateral US demonstrated multiple bilateral smooth or macrolobulated ovoid hypoechoic nodules (Figs. 4.5E–F).
- Breast MRI—Performed for problem-solving/preoperative exam, demonstrated highly suspicious, irregular, spiculated enhancing nodules consistent with carcinomata. (Patient declined additional MRI-guided biopsy before surgical excision.) right (Fig. 4.5G), left (Figs. 4.5H–K).

WORKUP

- Bilateral core biopsies were performed and demonstrated on the right (10:30), atypical cells; the left (12:30, 1:00), atypical papillary lesions.
- Bilateral excisional biopsies demonstrated invasive carcinoma, 2.4 cm, moderately differentiated (left); invasive cribriform carcinoma (right).
- She opted for bilateral mastectomies and sentinel node biopsy.

DISCUSSION

- When a patient is about to undergo excisional biopsy for an area of atypia demonstrated on core biopsy, consider performing a preoperative MRI, because it may suggest a definitive diagnosis.
- In addition, MRI may offer a more optimum method of obtaining definitive diagnosis before surgery, as well as show additional areas that need intervention. (This case is similar to case 2, in which MRI was done preoperatively for planned excisional biopsy of a discordant lesion.) Because MRI findings may be dramatically different from mammographic/sonographic findings, consider performing MRI for preoperative planning. Unfortunately, this patient did not want additional biopsy under MRI guidance, so underwent surgery twice.

• CASE 6

HISTORY

A 60-year-old woman who presented for evaluation of a right breast mass noted on CT, (Fig. 4.06A) during evaluation for a kidney mass. She denies any family history of breast or ovarian cancer. Prior screening mammograms had been negative.

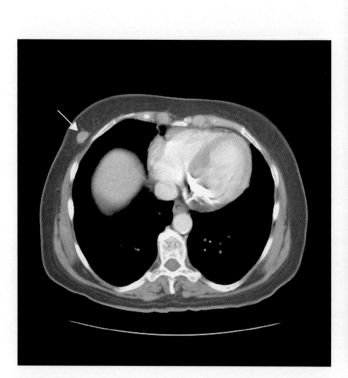

Figure 4.6A

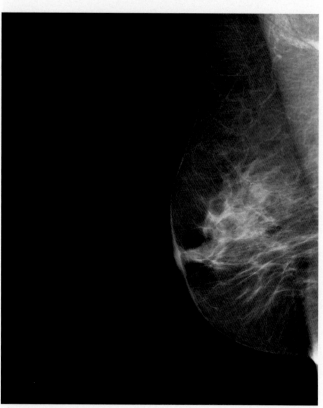

Figure 4.6B

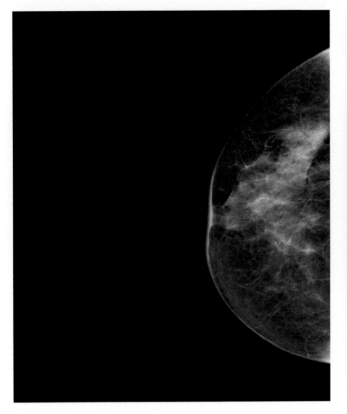

Figure 4.6C

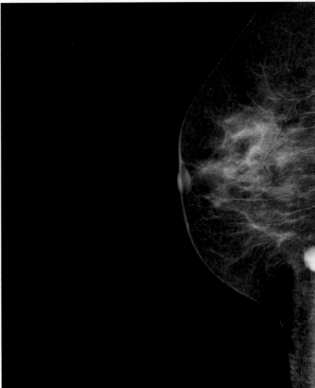

Figure 4.6D

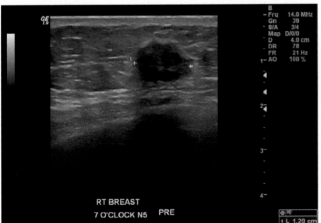

Figure 4.6E

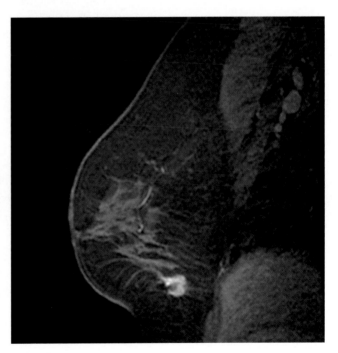

Figure 4.6F

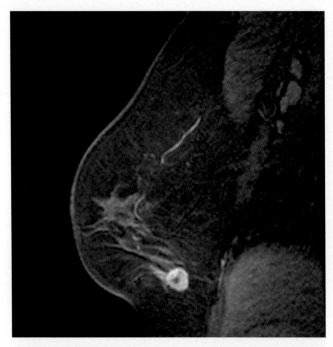

Figure 4.6G

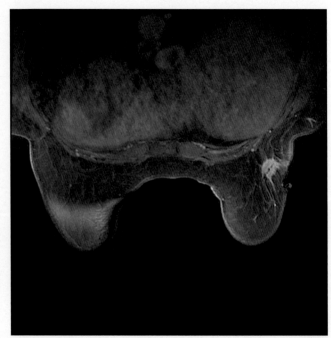

Figure 4.6H

FINDINGS

- CT (Fig. 4.6A)—Soft tissue mass R lower breast in subcutaneous tissue (arrow).
- Bilateral mammogram (right craniocaudal and mediolateral oblique views) were negative (Figs. 4.6B–C). An additional angulated view obtained later in workup revealed the anterior portion of a microlobulated mass, partially cut off the posterior edge of the film (Fig. 4.06D).
- Right US demonstrated a 14-mm solid nodule in the area of concern (Fig. 4.6E) (right outer lower quadrant).
- MRI, done for extent of disease evaluation, demonstrated a 1.5-cm, slightly irregular suspicious enhancing mass with mixed enhancement kinetics (Figs. 4.6F–H).

WORKUP

- US-guided core biopsy was consistent with an infiltrating duct adenocarcinoma.
- She underwent lumpectomy with sentinel node biopsy that revealed a 1.6-cm invasive ductal carcinoma with one positive sentinel node.

DISCUSSION

Although this patient was not high risk, she would have benefited from screening MRI because the lesion was too posterior (lower outer) to be consistently included on standard mammographic craniocaudal and mediolateral oblique views. Unfortunately, because of the extreme posterior location of her breast mass, this patient developed metastatic disease before breast cancer was detected on annual screening digital mammography.

• CASE 7

HISTORY

A 67-year-old woman presented with abnormal screening digital mammography. Her family history was positive for breast carcinoma, but did not meet the high-risk screening criteria and as a result had not been previously screened with MRI.

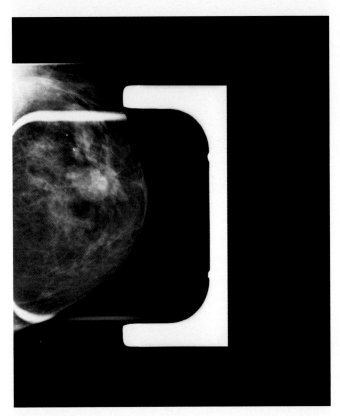

Figure 4.7A

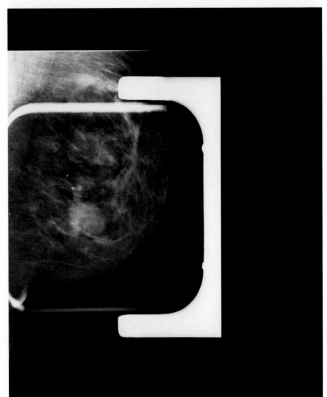

Figure 4.7B

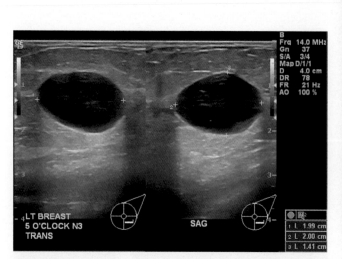

Figure 4.7C

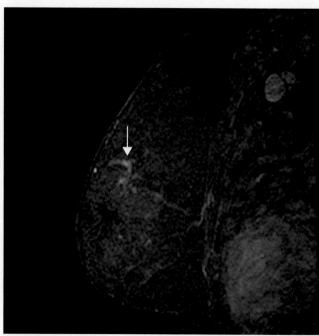

Figure 4.7D

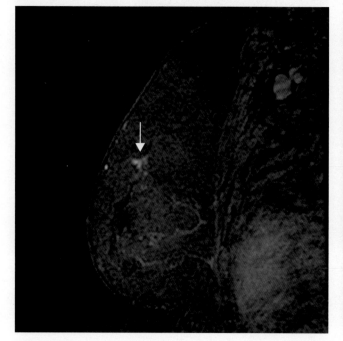

Figure 4.7E

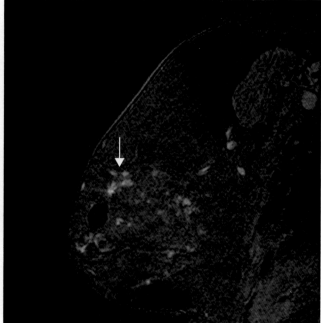

Figure 4.7F

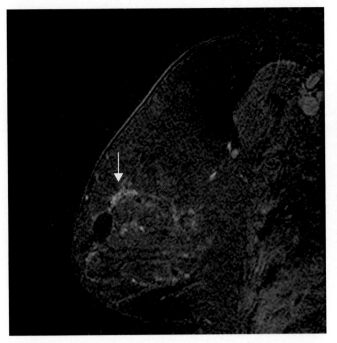

Figure 4.7G

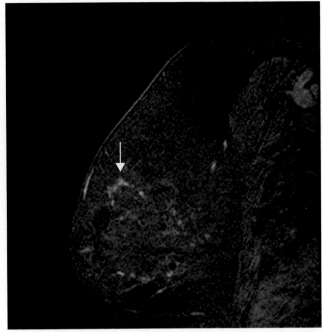

Figure 4.7H

FINDINGS

- Bilateral screening mammogram—Demonstrated new left mass and left architectural distortion (Figs. 4.7A–B).

- Left US—Demonstrated a large simple cyst (Fig. 4.7C). The area of distortion was thought to probably correspond to postsurgical scarring from a prior benign excisional biopsy.

- MRI was performed as mammographic problem solving, (to differentiate distortion caring from distortion from malignancy). Subtraction images (Figs. 4.7D–E) demonstrated grouped linear and branching enhancing foci in the 12:00 axis of the left breast. In addition, clumped nodular enhancement was noted in the right breast (Figs. 4.7F–H), 12:00 axis.

WORKUP

- Breast MRI core biopsies demonstrated the presence of left DCIS, right lobular carcinoma in situ.

- Patient underwent left lumpectomy and right excisional biopsy, which demonstrated extensive left high-grade DCIS and right lobular carcinoma in situ.

DISCUSSION

- We have had many patients who did not meet the cutoff for MRI screening (lifetime risk ≥20%), who have had MRI workup for clinical or imaging abnormalities that resulted in detection of a mammographically and clinically occult carcinoma. The American Cancer Society 2007 guidelines for high-risk MRI screening recommend that women with moderately elevated risk (15% to 20%) also consider MRI screening, and to make the decision on a case-by-case basis. Because this group of women is not usually being routinely screened with annual MRI, the yield of a single MRI demonstrating an occult malignancy is quite high in this group.

- Scar versus malignancy differentiation is not usually possible with digital mammography or sonography, but is usually easily distinguished on MRI.

• **Plate 1**

HISTORY

A 58-year-old woman with no risk factors presents with screening mammogram that demonstrated relatively fatty breasts with inconsistently seen patchy, asymmetric density in the right upper quadrant (Plates.4.1A–C). Her right US (Plate 4.1D) demonstrated a corresponding nonspecific mildly hypoechoic region. US core biopsy demonstrated atypia. MRI demonstrated a corresponding large irregular spiculated enhancing lesion (Plates 4.1E–H), with surrounding areas of linear enhancement. She underwent excisional biopsy, which demonstrated extensive DCIS. She subsequently underwent mastectomy with extensive residual DCIS noted.

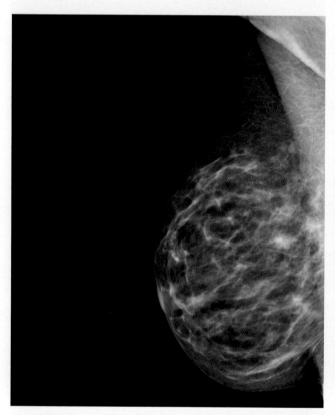

Plate 4.1A

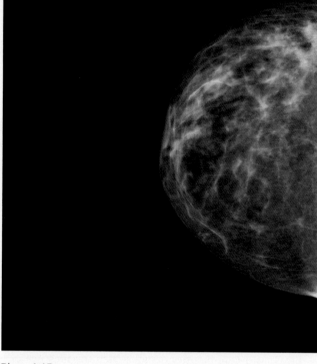

Plate 4.1B

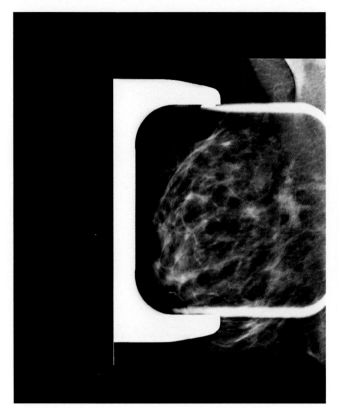

Plate 4.1C

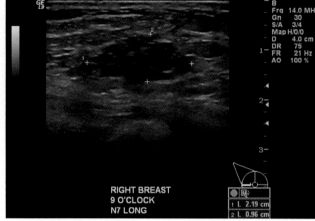

Plate 4.1D

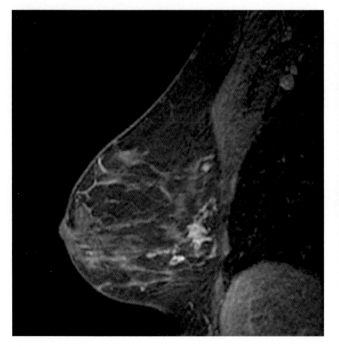

Plate 4.1E

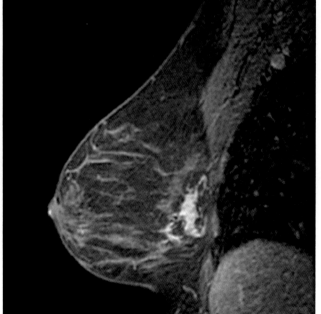

Plate 4.1F

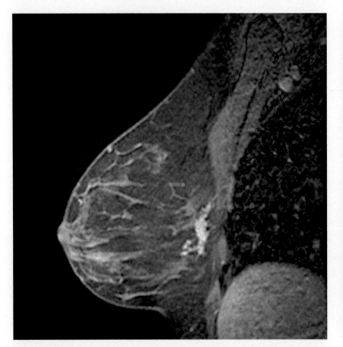

Plate 4.1G

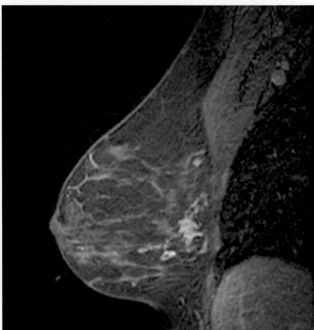

Plate 4.1H

DISCUSSION

Even in fatty breasts, malignancy can be relatively large and still be subtle or even occult on mammogram. Consider rebiopsy for an area of atypia with MRI guidance prior to surgical/excisional biopsy when level of suspicion of malignancy is high. Preoperative knowledge of the nature of the lesion will help the surgeon minimize number of surgical procedures.

• Plate 2

HISTORY

A 45-year-old woman who presents with a history of right nipple flattening/inversion for 2 months. She had a history of bilateral breast reduction 25 years ago without complication. Her risk factors include a sister with premenopausal breast cancer and first baby at age 40. She underwent a bilateral mammogram (baseline) and additional views were recommended for the left breast. She had not been getting high-risk MRI screening.

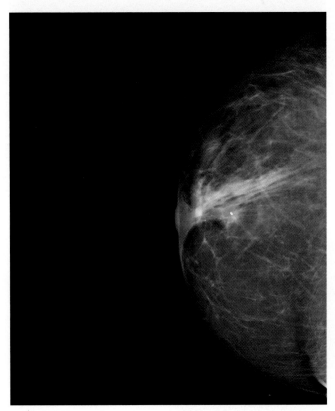

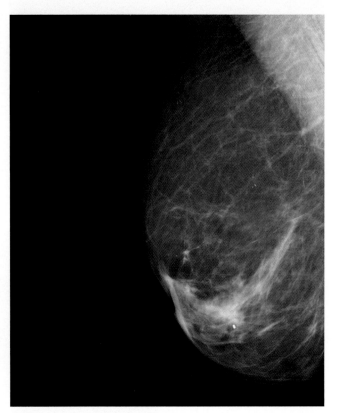

Plate 4.2A

Plate 4.2B

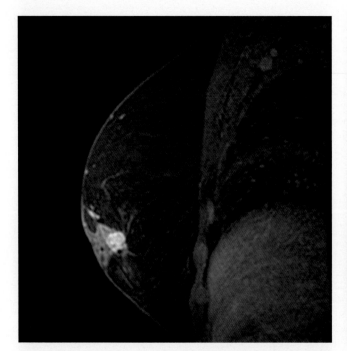

Plate 4.2C

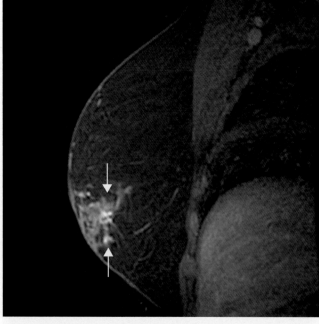

Plate 4.2D

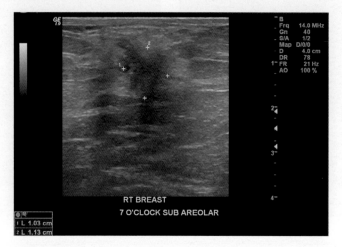

Plate 4.2E

FINDINGS

- Plates 4.2A–B—Right mammogram after biopsy demonstrated architectural changes related to her reduction. No abnormality had been appreciated on digital mammography prior to MRI.

- Plates 4.2C–D—Breast MRI, done for questionable mammographic *left* breast findings as well as unresolved clinical findings (nipple flattening) in the *right* breast— demonstrated an enhancing retroareolar *right* mass with small enhancing surrounding foci (Plates 4.2C–D), and adjacent linear spiculation extending inferiorly.

- Plate 4.2E—A targeted US was then performed and demonstrated a 1.1-cm spiculated hypoechoic area.

A core biopsy was performed and demonstrated a 9-mm invasive carcinoma, moderately to poorly differentiated, ER/PR+. She underwent lumpectomy with sentinel node biopsy. Final pathology revealed a 2.2-cm invasive ductal carcinoma with negative sentinel nodes.

DISCUSSION

Postsurgical changes from bilateral reduction surgery can limit visualization of even relatively large abnormalities on digital mammography and sonography. Detection of small breast cancers in this setting is hampered, and therefore MRI may be more sensitive in detecting early breast carcinomas in this group of patients.

• Plate 3

HISTORY

A 52-year-old woman who presents with routine screening digital mammography demonstrating a one view only finding of a new 1-cm vague density with mild distortion in the right inner posterior breast (Plates 4.3A–B). The area was unable to be definitively visualized on perpendicular views or on ultrasound. Problem-solving MRI scan (postcontrast and subtraction images) demonstrated a corresponding inner upper quadrant 1-cm faintly ring-enhancing spiculated lesion (Plates 4.2C–E). The kinetics are mixed (heterogeneous) predominantly progressive with areas of plateau kinetics (Plate 4.3F). Biopsy was recommended and subsequently performed with stereotactic guidance from a superior approach, which revealed invasive lobular carcinoma. She underwent lumpectomy with sentinel node biopsy. Final pathology revealed a 1.2-cm invasive pleomorphic lobular carcinoma with multiple positive nodes.

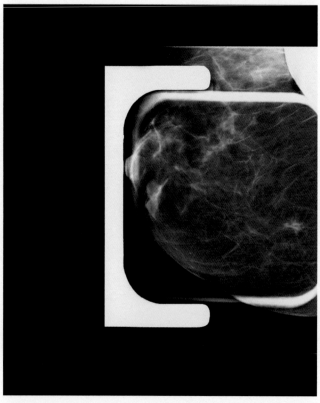

Plate 4.3A

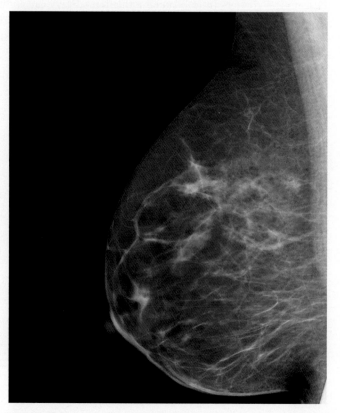

Plate 4.3B

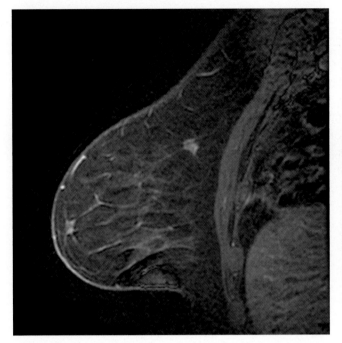

Plate 4.3C

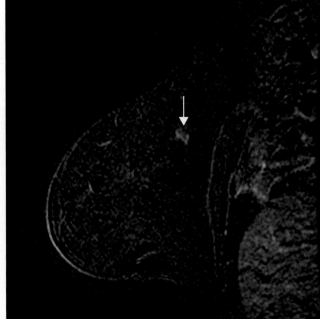

Plate 4.3D

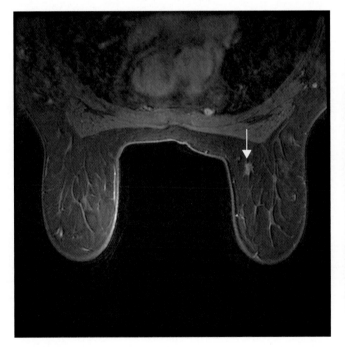

Plate 4.3E

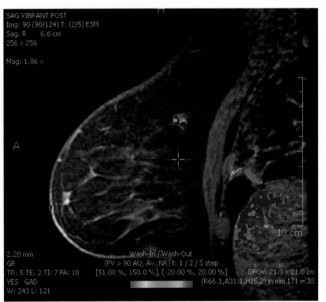

Plate 4.3F

DISCUSSION

- A common indication for problem-solving MRI is a one view only mammographic finding. Before MRI, these areas were often felt to be more likely parenchymal tissue and categorized as probably benign. Enhancing lesion corresponding to a one view finding/asymmetric density should be viewed with high suspicion.

- Lobular carcinomas can be difficult to detect on digital mammography and US. Although many are highly conspicuous on MRI, occasionally some demonstrate only low-level enhancement or fail to enhance completely.

- When a lesion cannot be localized in two views on digital mammography, MRI can localize the quadrant of the abnormality and, therefore, help plan the approach for stereotactic biopsy (or needle localization).

BENIGN LESIONS

• Plate 1

HISTORY

A 68-year-old woman asymptomatic with mass noted on routine digital mammography and confirmed on ultrasound and MRI.

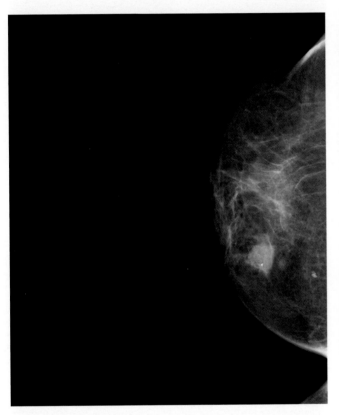

Plate 5.1A

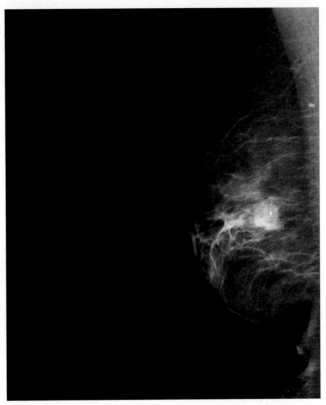

Plate 5.1B

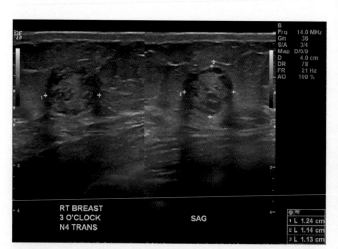

Plate 5.1C

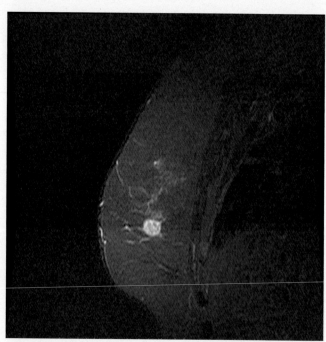

Plate 5.1D

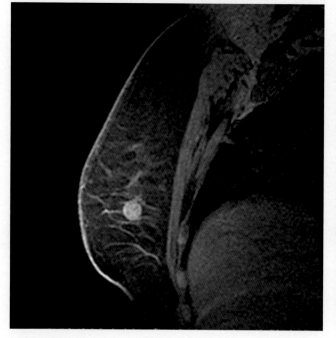

Plate 5.1E

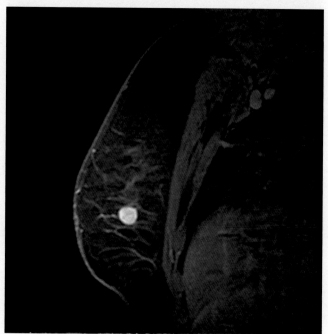

Plate 5.1F

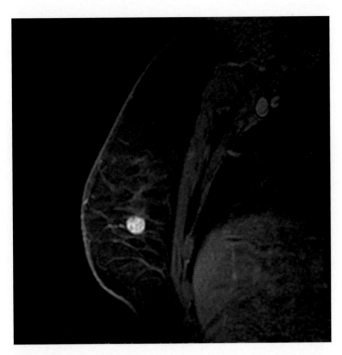

Plate 5.1G

FINDINGS

- Plates 5.1A–B—Digital mammography: Postbiopsy demonstrates a dominant mass with slightly indistinct margins.
- Plate 5.1C—Ultrasound (US): Demonstrates a complex rounded mass containing hyper and hypoechoic regions.
- Plates 5.1D–G—MRI: Demonstrates a relatively well-defined mass with high signal intensity on sagittal STIR images and progressive enhancement kinetics with heterogeneous central enhancement but margin remains sharp, even on delayed images. Although internal enhancement pattern varies from first series to last, no "blossoming" or increased size is seen.

DISCUSSION

The magnetic resonance imaging (MRI) appearance is similar to a fibroadenoma; however, the core biopsy result demonstrated suspicious atypical pathology and therefore excision as performed. Final pathology was myofibroblastoma.

The absense of "blossoming" size on delayed images favors benign etiology. This probably relates to the encapsulated native of certain benign nodules.

• Plate 2

HISTORY

A 44-year-old with positive family history of breast carcinoma undergoing high-risk MRI screening.

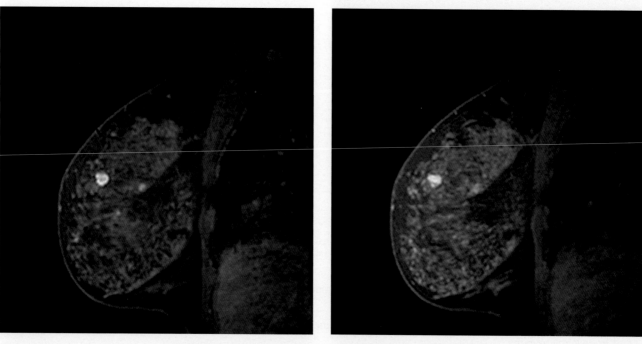

Plate 5.2A

Plate 5.2B

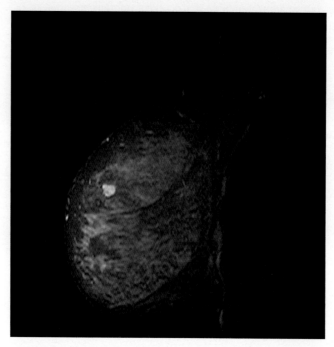

Plate 5.2C

FINDINGS

- Plate 5.2A—Sagittal STIR series demonstrating high-signal intensity.
- Plate 5.2B—First postcontrast series demonstrates a ring-enhancing lobulated 1-cm mass.
- Plate 5.2C—Last postcontrast series demonstrating progressive enhancement. Notice that although the enhancement is more intense and homogeneous ("filled in"), the borders of the lesion have not expanded or "blossomed," "blossoming" is a term we use to describe a finding more commonly associated with malignancy.

DISCUSSION

Final pathology on MRI-guided core biopsy was fibroadenoma. MRI-guided core biopsy was recommended because of suspicion associated with ring enhancement and slightly irregular border. However, benign features noted include progressive enhancement and bright images on sagittal STIRs. Benign and malignant lesions can share some features. It is important to consider the entire picture before deciding on concordance of the pathology and imaging. This did not require surgical excision and was stable on 6-month postbiopsy follow-up. Also in the differential diagnosis is papilloma. Papillary lesions enhance very intensely. As a result, many more papillomas are detected on MRI as compared with digital mammography.

• Plate 3

HISTORY

A 60-year-old woman with a newly diagnosed carcinoma for which MRI was performed, for extent of disease evaluation. On the contralateral side, a characteristically benign lesion was noted, for which no intervention is required.

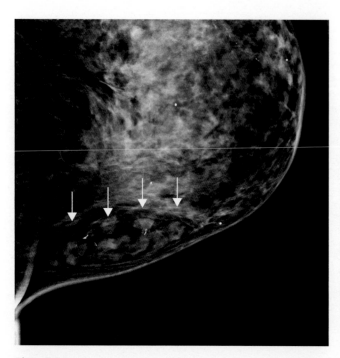

Plate 5.3A

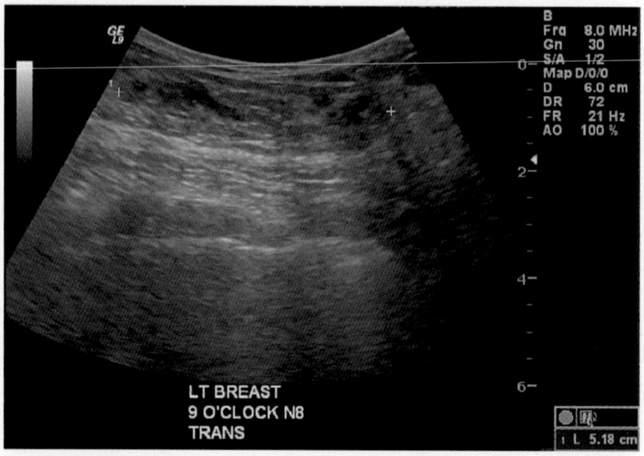

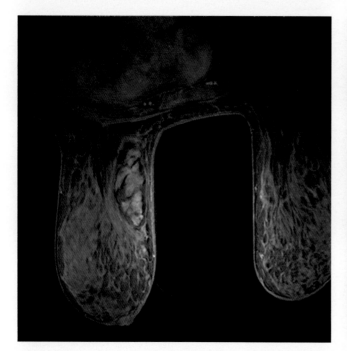

Plate 5.3B

Plate 5.3C

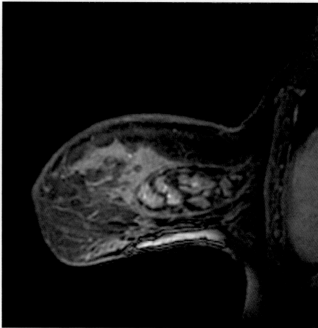

Plate 5.3D

FINDINGS

- Plate 5.3A—Mammogram demonstrates the typical "sausage slice," mottled appearance of this well-circumscribed fat-containing mass.
- Plate 5.3B—US demonstrates a well-circumscribed margin with internal hypoechoic and hyperechoic areas corresponding to fatty (hypoechoic) and glandular (hyperechoic) elements.
- Plates 5.3C–D—MRI demonstrates a corresponding lesion with similar "sausage slice" appearance, containing mixed fatty and fibroglandular elements.

DISCUSSION

This lesion is a typical "Aunt Minnie" visibly different from the surrounding tissue but not requiring any intervention or diagnosis. The feature of hamartoma or fibroadenolipoma is as apparent and characteristic on MRI as they are on digital mammography.

• **Plate 4**

HISTORY

A 39-year-old woman who presents for high-risk screening MRI and history of benign excisional biopsy.

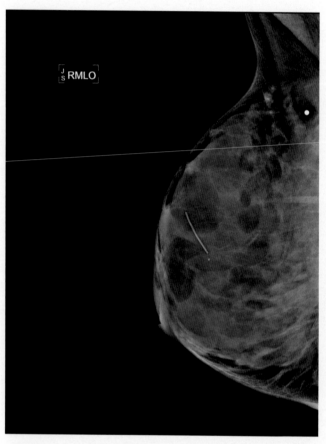

Plate 5.4A

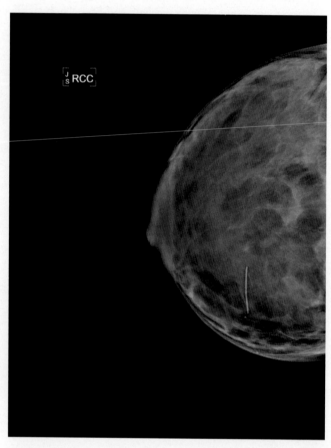

Plate 5.4B

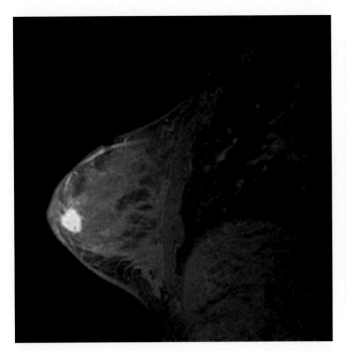

Plate 5.4C

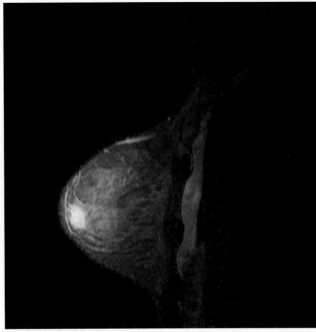

Plate 5.4D

FINDINGS

- Plates 5.4A–B—Screening digital mammography demonstrates dense breasts.
- Plates 5.4C–D—MRI demonstrates a smooth progressively enhancing, retroareolar mass that is bright on sagittal STIR images (Plate P5.4D).

DISCUSSION

These features are similar to fibroadenoma, but biopsy was recommended because of large size and high-risk status. Final pathology was hemangioma.

Papillomata, fibroadenomas, hemangioma, and myofibroblastomas all share common features of enhancement kinetics that are more usually progressive, morphologic features of smooth, well-defined margins, and usually high intensity on STIR (or T2) series.

• Plate 5

HISTORY

A 63-year-old woman with MRI was performed for extent of disease evaluation. These images demonstrate the typical appearance of an inflamed or complex cyst.

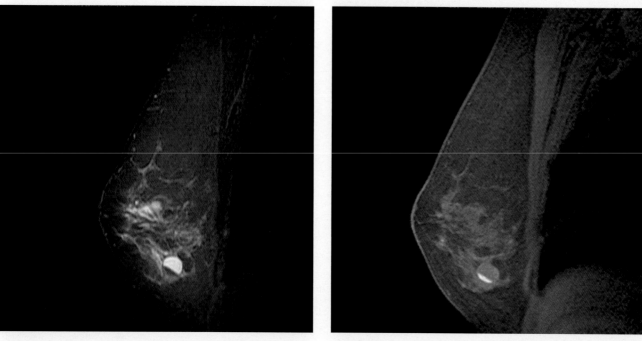

Plate 5.5A

Plate 5.5B

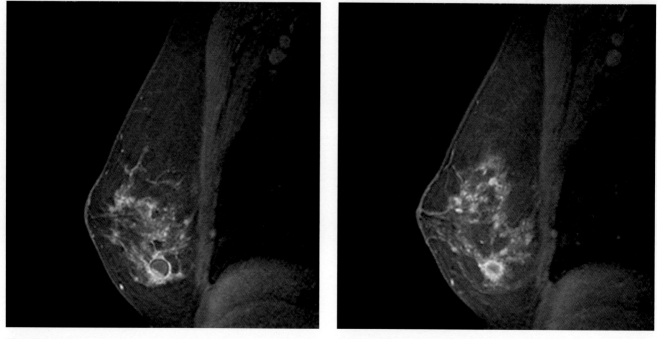

Plate 5.5C

Plate 5.5D

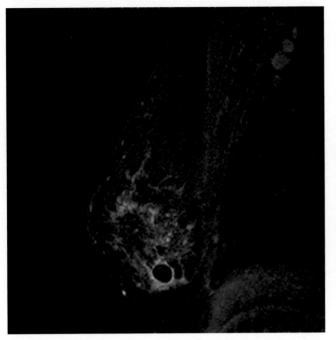

Plate 5.5E

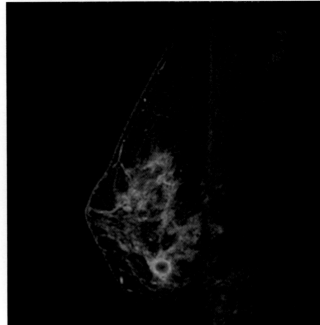

Plate 5.5F

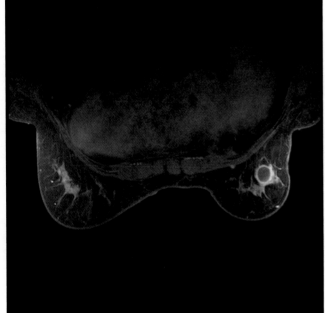

Plate 5.5G

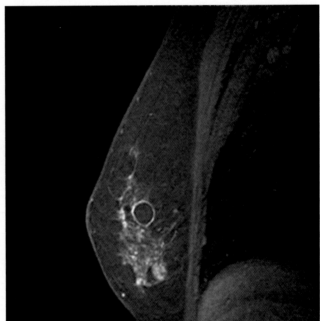

Plate 5.5H

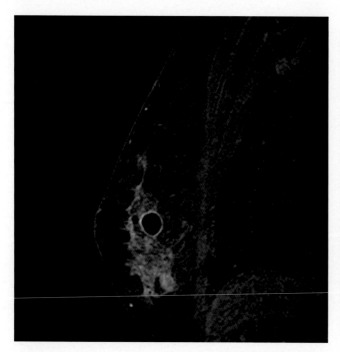

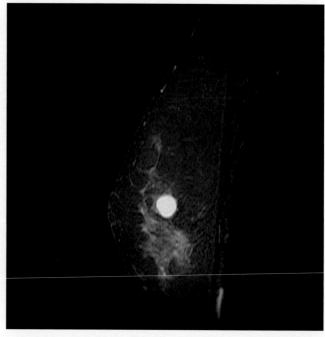

Plate 5.5I   Plate 5.5J

FINDINGS

- Plate 5.5A—Sagittal STIR image demonstrates simple fluid component superiorly with debris inferiorly.
- Plate 5.5B—Demonstrates precontrast images with hemorrhagic or proteinaceous debris inferiorly.
- Plates 5.5C–D—Postcontrast image demonstrating slightly thick and irregular rim enhancement.
- Plates 5.5E–F—Subtraction series.
- Plate 5.5G—Axial series.
- Plates 5.5H–J—Demonstrate in the same patient, a typical simple cyst with more common thinner, more uniform rim enhancement, and homogenous high-intensity on sagittal STIRs. Most simple cysts do not demonstrate any enhancement.

DISCUSSION

Rim enhancement is not uncommon with cysts, but when inflamed, the rim enhancement can be thicker and more irregular and as a result be difficult to distinguish from ring enhancement of a carcinoma. In this case, the sharp internal margin surrounding the fluid component suggests the benign nature of this lesion. US may help, but may also demonstrate similar features of a complex cyst, and aspiration may be warranted depending on the clinical setting.

• Plate 6

HISTORY

A 55-year-old woman status postbilateral reduction mammoplasty with abnormal digital mammography and sonography, unable to exclude mass because of scarring and postsurgical changes.

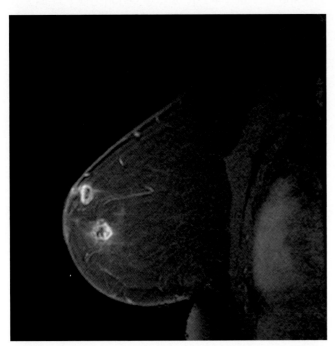

Plate 5.6A

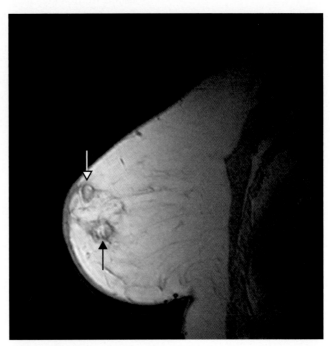

Plate 5.6B

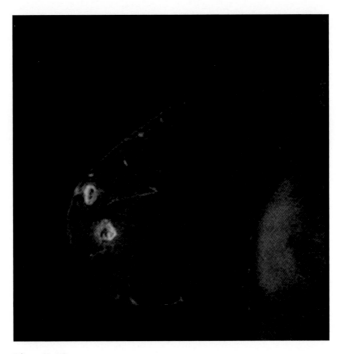

Plate 5.6C

FINDINGS

- Plates 5.6A–C—Demonstrates two ring-enhancing lesions that are demonstrated to contain fat on the nonfat suppressed series (Fig. 5.6B).

DISCUSSION

Central fat intensity on non-fat-suppressed series is diagnostic of fat necrosis. Without the non-fat-suppressed series, biopsy may be needed to distinguish these ring-enhancing lesions from malignancy. It takes approximately 1.5 minutes to perform the non-fat-suppressed series, and we routinely do this specifically for this purpose. Fat necrosis can be postsurgery (e.g., lumpectomy, reduction, mammoplasty, benign biopsy) or posttrauma, and is especially common in Transverse Rectus Abdominis Myocutaneous (TRAM) flap reconstructions (see Plate 7). If fat cannot be demonstrated centrally, biopsy should be performed to rule out malignancy, unless fat necrosis can be confirmed definitely for that specific lesion by mammographic features.

• Plate 7

HISTORY

A 52-year-old woman after mastectomy with TRAM flap reconstruction for extensive DCIS.

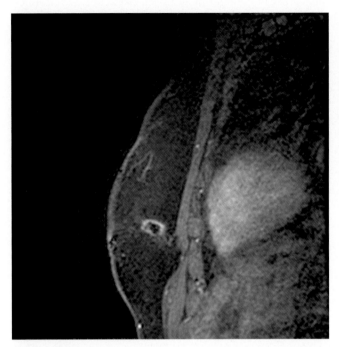

Plate 5.7A

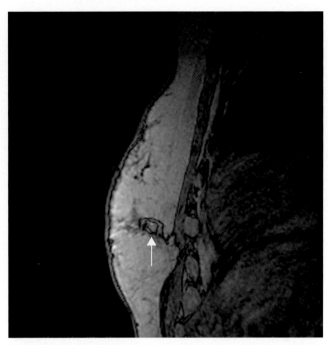

Plate 5.7B

FINDINGS

- Plates 5.7A–B—Postcontrast and non-fat-suppressed series demonstrating another example of fat necrosis.

• Plate 8

HISTORY

A 63-year-old postradiation and lumpectomy patient who developed multiple areas of fat necrosis, some of which are palpable. Because of some questionable imaging features and prominent clinical findings, core biopsy of the right inner upper quadrant was performed and demonstrated fat necrosis.

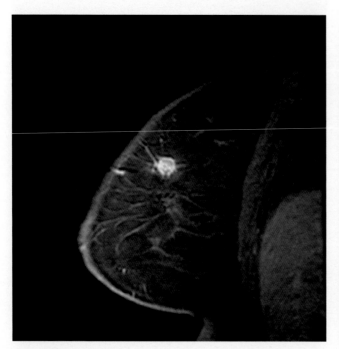

Plate 5.8A

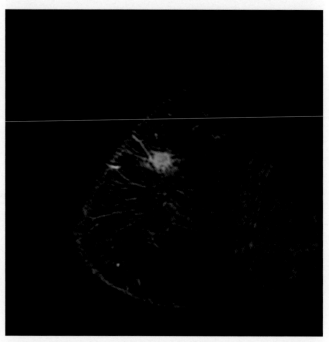

Plate 5.8B

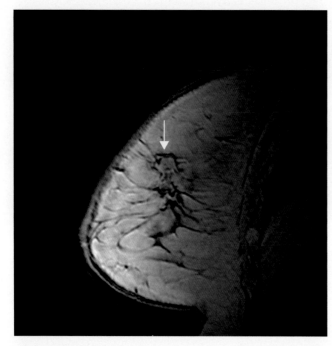

Plate 5.8C

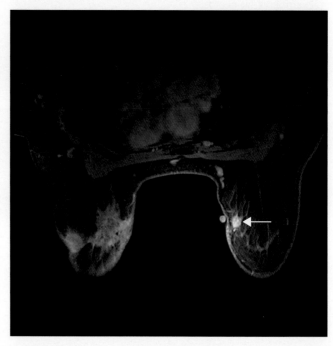

Plate 5.8D

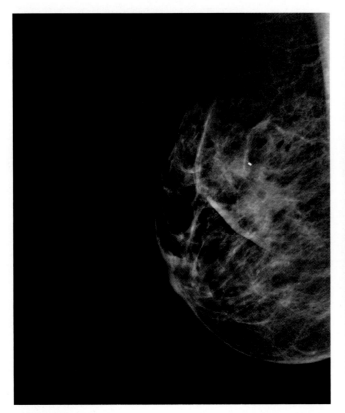

Plate 5.8E

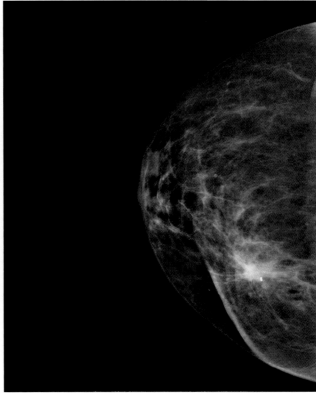

Plate 5.8F

FINDINGS

- Plates 5.8A–B—Post contrast & subtraction series demonstrate an enhancing spiculated max.
- Plate 5.8C—Non-fat suppressed series demonstrates the mass to be composed of fat intensity material.
- Plate 5.8D—Axial series with vitamin E capsule over the palpable lump.
- Postcontrast subtraction, non-fat-suppressed, and axial MRI scans Plates 5.8(A–D). Note the vitamin E capsule placed over the palpable lump on the axial image.
- Mammographic images obtained after core biopsy with clip placement (Plates 5.8E–F).

DISCUSSION

The larger fat necrosis lesions, usually, (but not always) can be seen to contain fat on the non-fat-suppressed series and therefore do not require biopsy. The smaller ones and occasionally some of the larger lesions (especially earlier in their course of development) may not demonstrate internal fat and therefore should be evaluated with core biopsy. Some patients have a greater tendency to form fat necrosis, and will continue to form additional areas of involvement on serial exams.

• Plate 9

HISTORY

A 42-year-old woman with a palpable axillary tail mass. US-guided core biopsy was requested but no abnormal area could be visualized sonographically. Patient was scheduled for surgical biopsy. She underwent MRI as a preoperative and clinical problem-solving exam.

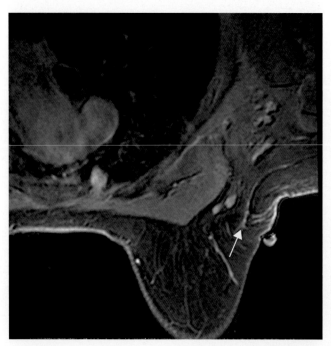

Plate 5.9A

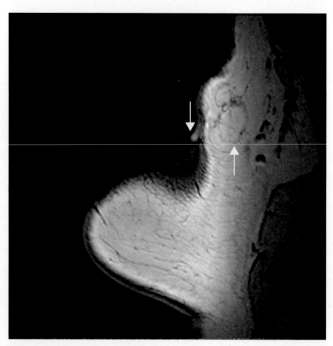

Plate 5.9B

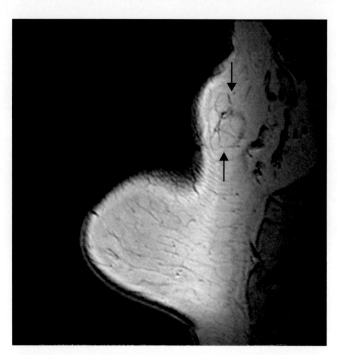

Plate 5.9C

FINDINGS

- Plate 5.9A—Axial image with vitamin E capsule are palpable lump demonstrate only fat intensity tissue, suggestion of thin capsule, and normal appearing underlying axillary nodes.
- Plates 5.9B–C—Non-fat suppressed sagittal series demonstrates thinly encapsulated, purely fatty tumor corresponding to palpable "lump" marker.

DISCUSSION

For MRI, a vitamin E capsule was placed over the palpable lump. On all sequences, including non-fat-suppressed, the palpable abnormality corresponded to a thinly encapsulated fatty tumor with signal intensity identical to other areas of adipose tissue. This is consistent with a lipoma. Lipomas tend to be nonenhancing, large, oval, thinly encapsulated fatty masses. These are characteristically benign and do not require further follow-up. Excision however may be performed for cosmetic reasons.

• Plate 10

HISTORY

A 50-year-old woman undergoing annual high-risk screening MRI.

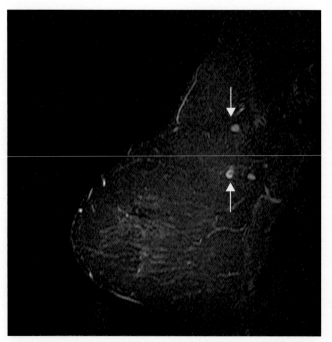

Plate 5.10A

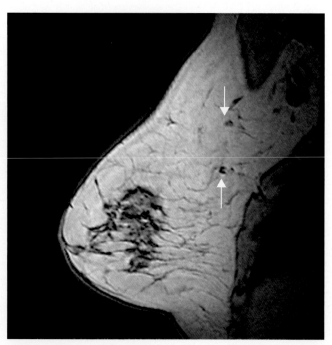

Plate 5.10B

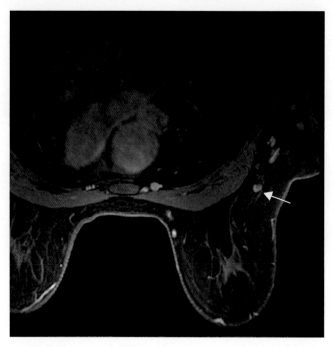

Plate 5.10C

FINDINGS

- Sagittal STIR series demonstrates small high intensity axillary nodes. (Plate 5.10A).
- Non-fat suppressed series demonstrates central/hilar fat. (Plate 5.10B).
- Axial series demonstrates characterstic "C" shape. (Plate 5.10C).
- STIR, non-fat-suppressed and axial images. The "C" shape or "donut" shape characteristic of a benign lymph node may only be apparent on one series, so check all series for the morphologic features.

DISCUSSION

These images demonstrate characteristic appearance of lymph nodes in the breast and axilla. These are seen as round to oval intensely enhancing small nodules, but are nearly always easily differentiated from malignancy by certain features. They tend to be C-shaped (or kidney bean-shaped with hilum), bright on sagittal STIR, usually hanging off or in close proximity to a vessel (like a grape on a stem), and may contain central fat (if large enough) on non-fat-suppressed series. However, they demonstrate suspicious wash out kinetics, which may even be more intense than most cancers. They can occur in any quadrant of the breast, but are most frequent in the upper outer quadrant. In the axilla, lymph nodes can be very large (>2 cm) but still be benign, as long as the cortex is thin relative to the fatty center/hilum.

• Plate 11

HISTORY

A 35-year-old woman presented with abnormal MRI done for high-risk screening (positive family history), MRI demonstrated a large smooth oval progressively enhancing mass with some nonenhancing internal septations and high signal intensity on sagittal STIR. These findings suggest a fibroadenoma, but should be confirmed with needle biopsy, especially in a high-risk patient and a lesion of this size (>2 cm).

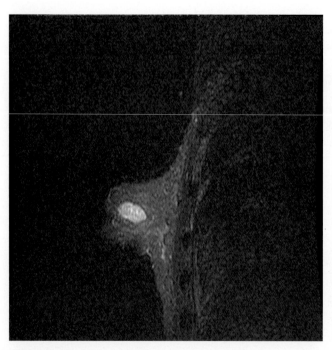

Plate 5.11A

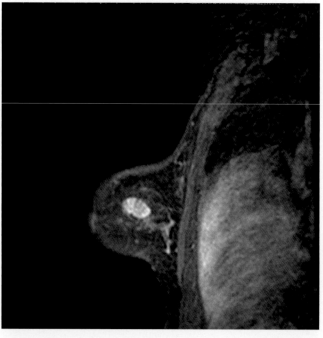

Plate 5.11B

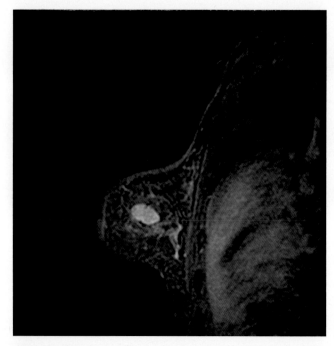

Plate 5.11C

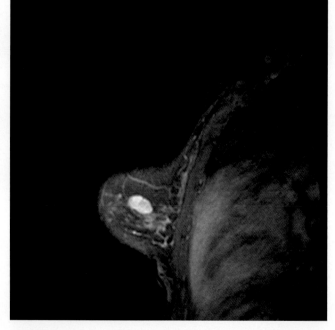

Plate 5.11D

FINDINGS

- Plate 5.11A—STIR series demonstrates high signal intensity and smooth borders.
- Plate 5.11B—1st post contrast series demonstrates enhancement.
- Plate 5.11C—Subtraction series.
- Plate 5.11D—Last post contrast series demonstrates progressive enhancement.
- Postcontrast first and fourth, subtraction, and STIR scans demonstrate the large smooth oval progressively enhancing mass.
- Note that this benign lesion does not appear to increase in size (blossom) on more delayed images. The margin is as sharp and well defined on the last postcontrast series as on the first.

DISCUSSION

Many fibroadenomas enhance, and therefore must be biopsied, to differentiate from a smoothly circumscribed carcinoma. Features that suggest this benign diagnosis include smooth sharp margin on all series, high intensity on sagittal STIR, progressive enhancement, and nonenhancing internal septations. Occasionally, if these lesions are small and meet the above criteria, or there are biopsy proven similar appearing fibroadenomata elsewhere in the breasts, these lesions may be closely followed instead of biopsied, to confirm stability/benign nature.

• CASE 1

HISTORY

A 45-year-old woman with asymmetric nodular tissue containing loosely grouped calcifications in the right lower breast on mammogram, that had been present for 5 years, but now appeared increased in size and density.

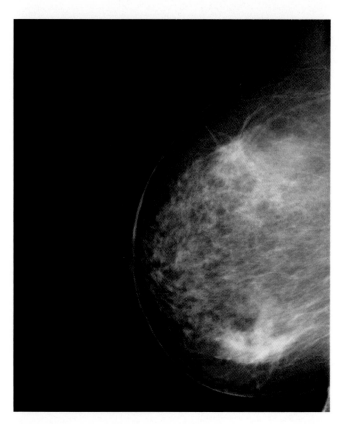

Figure 6.1A

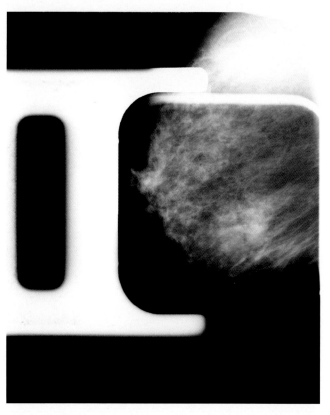

Figure 6.1B

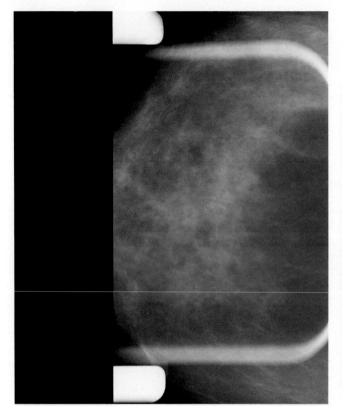

Figure 6.1C

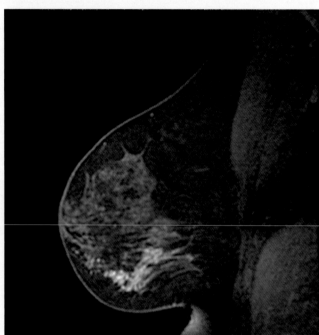

Figure 6.1D

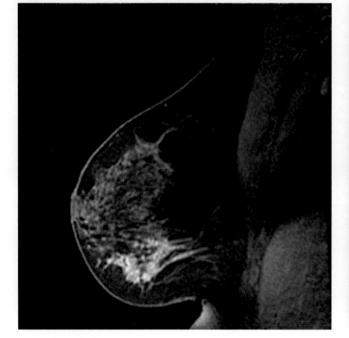

Figure 6.1E

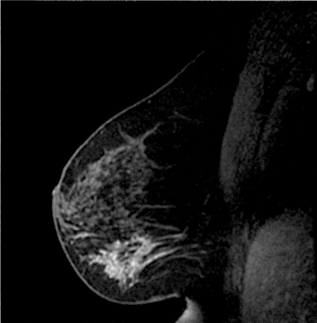

Figure 6.1F

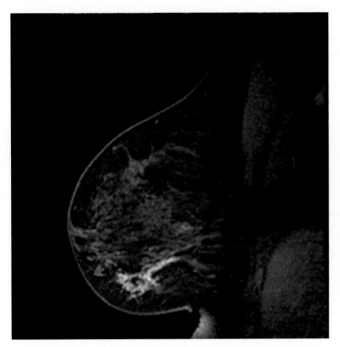

Figure 6.1G

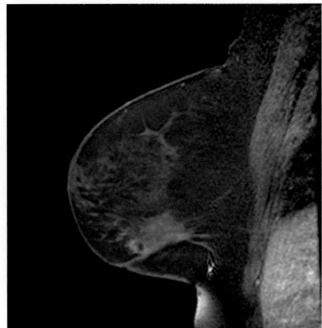

Figure 6.1H

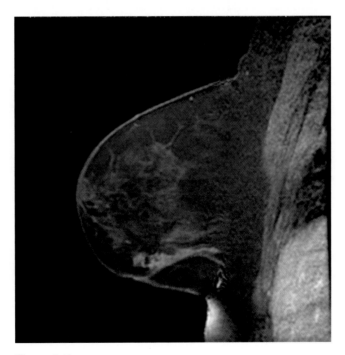

Figure 6.1I

FINDINGS

- Figures 6.1A–C—Mammographic images (lateral, spot compression, and magnification) demonstrating a large nodular asymmetric density with microcalcifications in the 6:00 axis, thought to have increased from prior exams.
- Figures 6.1D–G—Sagittal postcontrast magnetic resonance imaging (MRI) scans demonstrating a large area of clumped and linear enhancement along 6:00 axis in a segmental distribution with spiculation and distortion, very suspicious in appearance.
- Figures 6.1H–I—Postcontrast sagittal images 2 years later (after excision) demonstrating no significant residual enhancement. Nonenhancing postoperative changes are noted.

WORKUP

- Ultrasound (US) was negative.
- She underwent MRI for mammographic problem solving. MRI demonstrated suspicious segmental and clumped enhancement spanning over a 5-cm region. A stereotactic needle biopsy was done and pathology revealed atypical ductal hyperplasia. Patient went to surgery for excisional biopsy with wire localization. Because of the highly suspicious appearance on MRI, two wires were used during localization to bracket the area for excision. Final path demonstrated extensive atypical ductal hyperplasia. Multiple postsurgical MRIs have been obtained for follow-up.

DISCUSSION

MRI is very sensitive. High-risk lesions can appear as suspicious as cancers. One of the early concerns about using MRI was high sensitivity and low specificity. However, despite the overlap in appearance between some benign lesions and malignancy, our positive predictive value with MRI is as good or better than our positive predictive value in digital mammography, and significantly better than our positive predictive values in US. Also, we have found that more of our MRI false positive cases are associated with high-risk lesions than our false-positive mammographic/sonographic biopsies. This suggests that although there is an equivalent false-positive rate with MRI and digital mammography, the MRI false positives may have mere clinical relevance than some of the mammographic false positives.

• **CASE 2**

HISTORY

A 47-year-old woman presented with abnormal screening mammogram, with architectural distortion in the 12:00 axis of the right breast.

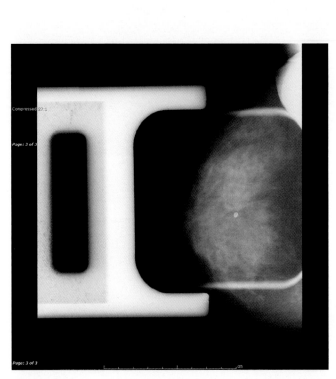

Figure 6.2A

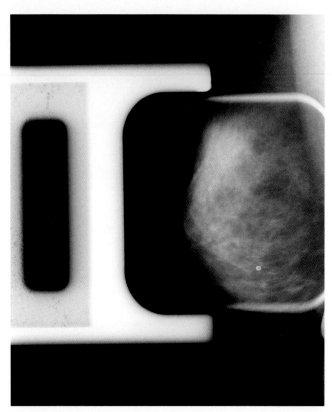

Figure 6.2B

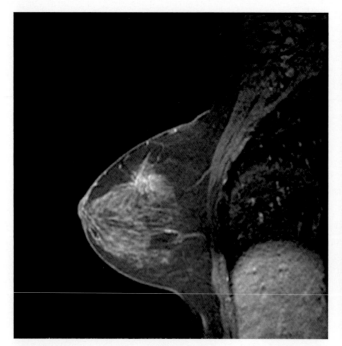

Figure 6.2C

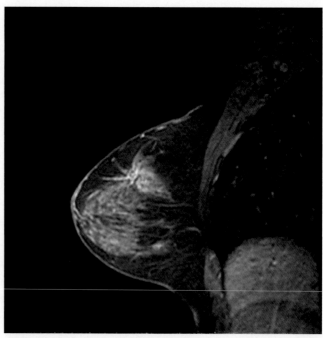

Figure 6.2D

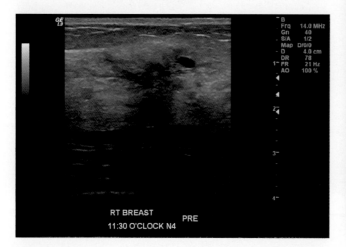

Figure 6.2E

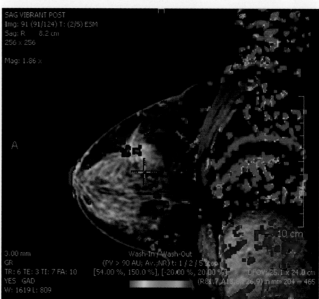

Figure 6.2F

FINDINGS

- Figures 6.2A–B—Spot views from digital mammogram demonstrating dense breast parenchyma and architectural distortion in the 12:00 axis.
- Figures 6.2C–D—Postcontrast sagittal MRI images demonstrating a large spiculated faintly enhancing area of architectural distortion. This appearance is quite suspicious, especially for lobular carcinomas.
- Figure 6.2E—Targeted US demonstrating hypoechoic shadowing thought to correspond to the abnormal area on MRI.
- Figures 6.2F—Color kinetic analysis demonstrates low-level progressive enhancement. Although these kinetics suggest a benign etiology, they can be seen in some invasive lobular carcinomas. The suspicious morphology (spiculation/distortion) makes biopsy necessary.

WORKUP

- MRI was obtained as mammographic problem solving and demonstrated a lesion with faintly enhancing radiating spicules and architectural distortion, with no history of biopsy. This was considered suspicious.
- A targeted US was performed and an area of shadowing was seen, believed to correspond to MRI and mammographic findings.
- A core biopsy was done, which demonstrated atypical ductal hyperplasia. The patient underwent excisional biopsy (with MRI localization). Final pathology demonstrated florid atypical ductal hyperplasia. She has been subsequently followed with digital mammography and MRI and has no further suspicious findings.

DISCUSSION

As in the previous case, areas of atypical ductal hyperplasia (ADH) can appear very suspicious on MRI, and needle biopsy and excision are indicated. Although these suspicious areas may prove to represent false-positive lesions (e.g., atypical hyperplasia or lobular carcinoma in situ [LCIS]) knowledge of these high-risk lesions can impact a patient's long-term surveillance and treatment.

Targeted US is a study frequently performed after MRI. This should still be considered even if a recent US had been performed and was negative. US scanning is less reproducible and is more operator dependent than other imaging modalities. Although most radiologists who interpret MRI are familiar with concept of targeted or second look (repeat) US, patients and referring physicians are not. In this case, US had been performed prior to MRI, but lesion was not seen until the second look. Because US is relatively inexpensive, not uncomfortable (no compression) and uses no radiation or contrast, there is very little downside to performing a repeat study, However, the absence of findings on second look US should never preclude follow-up of suspicious MRI findings, because approximately 50% of MRI findings will not be visible on US.

• CASE 3

HISTORY

A 37-year-old woman who presented with an abnormal mammogram and strongly positive family history. She was recalled from screening mammogram for questionable architectural distortion in the right upper outer quadrant.

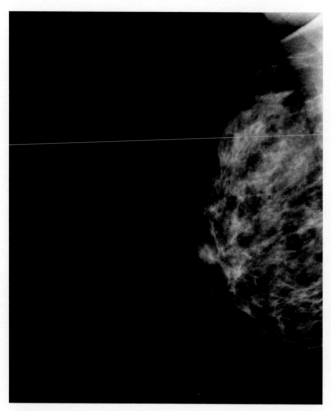

Figure 6.3A

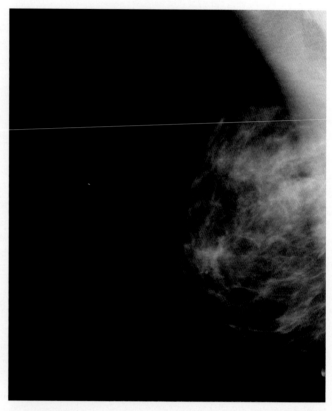

Figure 6.3B

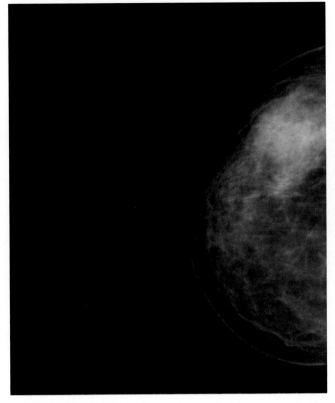

Figure 6.3C

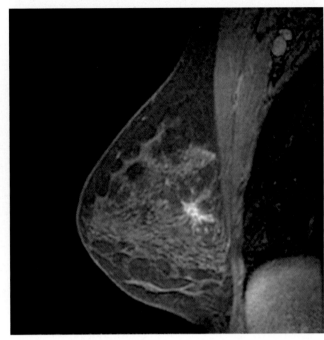

Figure 6.3D

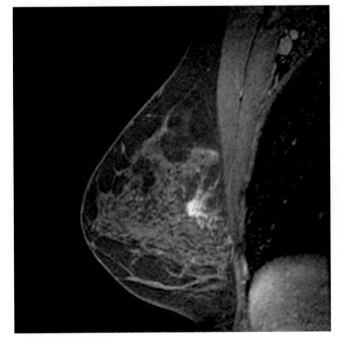

Figure 6.3E

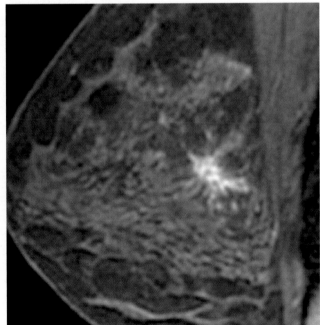

Figure 6.3F

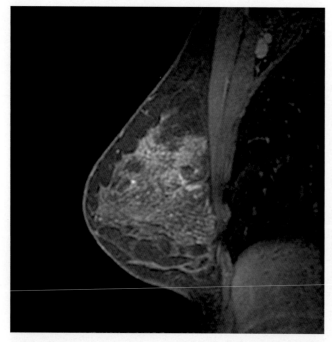

Figure 6.3G

Figure 6.3H

FINDINGS

- Figures 6.3A–C—Digital mammogram images demonstrating heterogeneously dense parenchyma and questionable inconsistently seen right upper quadrant distortion.
- Figures 6.3D–E—Sagittal postcontrast images demonstrating a spiculated enhancing mass in the posterior aspect of the right breast.
- Figure 6.3F—Magnified image with radiating spicules.
- Figure 6.3G—3 months after surgery, MRI through the same region demonstrating no residual mass and mild postsurgical changes.
- Figure 6.3H—This spiculated area demonstrates mixed plateau and progressive enhancement kinetics. Biopsy was recommended based on highly suspicious morphology. (color enhanced kinetic analysis)

WORKUP

- On additional views, this area persisted but no corresponding abnormality was seen on US. MRI was performed as mammographic problem solving ('one view only' finding). Sagittal postcontrast series demonstrated an irregular, spiculated, enhancing mass in the posterior breast along the 9:00 axis. MRI core biopsy was performed and demonstrated atypical ductal hyperplasia. Surgical biopsy was performed and demonstrated florid ductal hyperplasia, and no atypia. Because of the highly suspicious appearance on MRI and absence of concordant findings on pathology, MRI was repeated 3 months after surgery. No residual enhancement was seen.

DISCUSSION

This is an unusual case in that a lesion with highly suspicious features on MRI such as this, usually is found to be malignant. If a lesion looks this suspicious, and pathology is benign, perform a follow-up scan to ensure the area of concern was adequately biopsied/removed.

• CASE 4

HISTORY

A 60-year-old woman with positive family history of breast cancer presents for her high-risk screening MRI. Her bilateral mammogram was normal and demonstrated fatty breasts. Her MRI demonstrated minimal background enhancement with a focal area of faint clumped enhancement and grouped ("clustered") progressively enhancing foci.

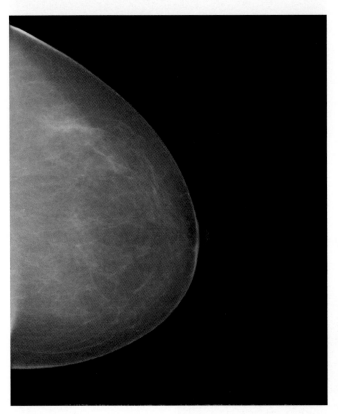

Figure 6.4A

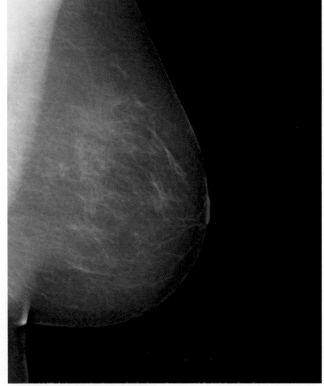

Figure 6.4B

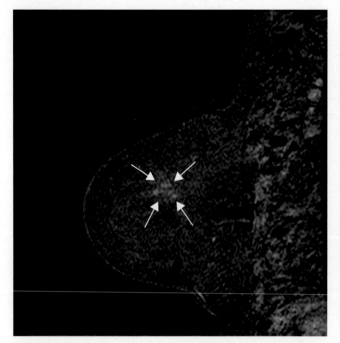

Figure 6.4C

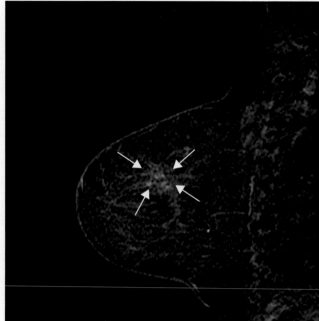

Figure 6.4D

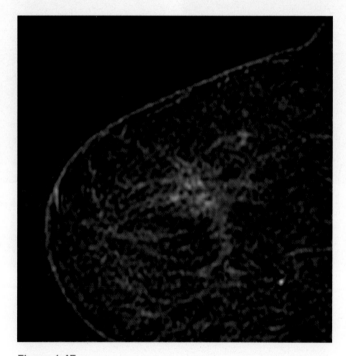

Figure 6.4E

FINDINGS

- Figures 6.4A–B—Digital mammogram demonstrating fatty breast parenchyma without abnormality.
- Figures 6.4C–D—Demonstrates subtracted images with grouped foci of enhancement. In Figure 6.4D, there is questionable mild distortion (left upper outer quadrant).
- Figure 6.4E—Demonstrates magnified images showing faint progressive grouped enhancing foci with mild distortion.

WORKUP

- Because this area was the ONLY enhancing region in the entire exam, MRI core biopsy was recommended. This demonstrated LCIS. Surgical excision demonstrated more extensive LCIS as well as micro invasive lobular carcinoma.

DISCUSSION

This area would not have been easily distinguished in a breast with more significant background enhancement. Generally, LCIS shows non-masslike enhancement or grouped enhancing foci. It can also have a linear enhancement pattern, similar to DCIS. When an area of enhancing foci are grouped or "clustered" like this, be suspicious, because it may represent DCIS. Although this area represented LCIS, the presence of multiple foci of microinvasion made this lesion highly significant!

• CASE 5

HISTORY

A 43-year-old woman with a strongly positive family history for breast cancer undergoing her baseline high-risk MRI screening, which demonstrated a left lower inner quadrant area of clumped enhancement and grouped enhancing foci arranged in a segmental distribution and associated with mild distortion.

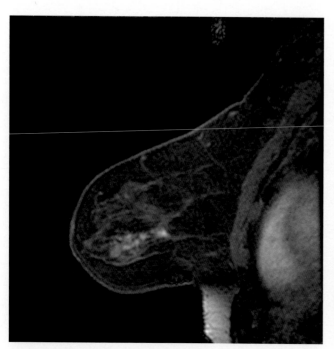

Figure 6.5A

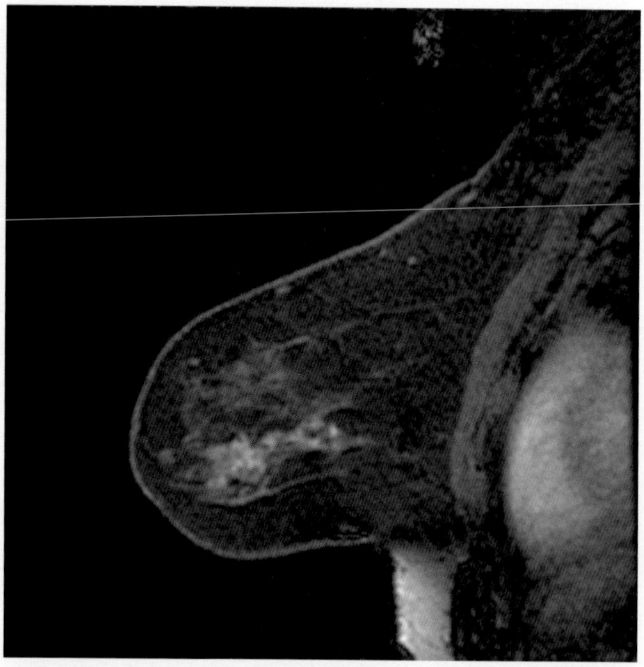

Figure 6.5B

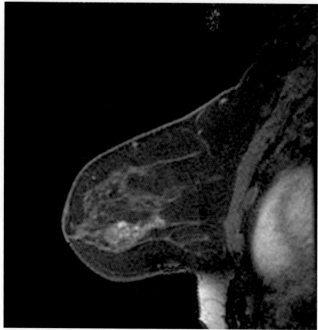

Figure 6.5C

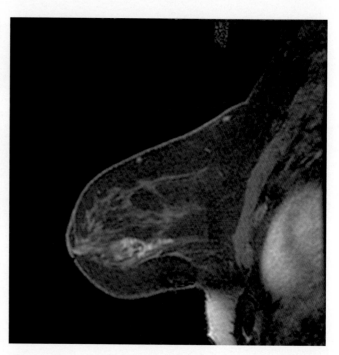

Figure 6.5D

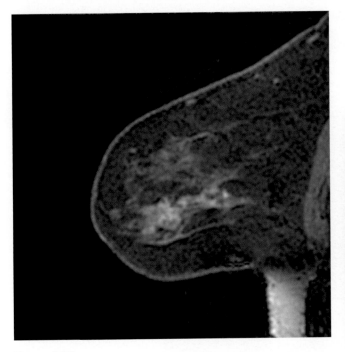

Figure 6.5E

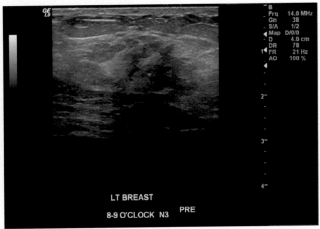

Figure 6.5F

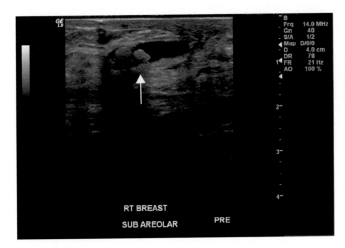

Figure 6.5G

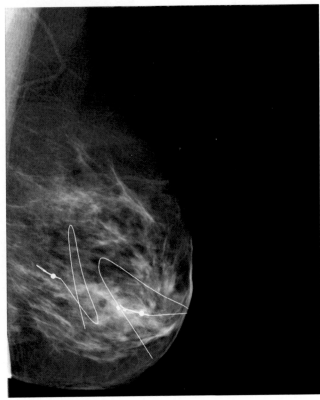

Figure 6.5H

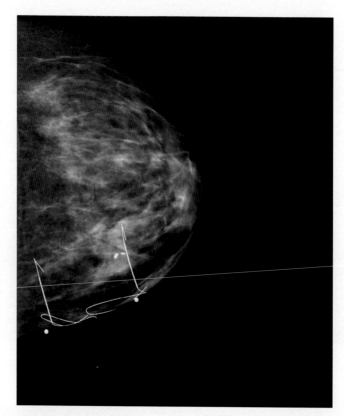

Figure 6.5I

FINDINGS

- Figures 6.5A–D—Sagittal postcontrast MRI images demonstrating a large area of segmental clumped enhancement and clustered enhancing foci arranged in a ductal/segmental pattern.
- Figure 6.5E—Demonstrates a magnified image showing mild distortion.
- Figure 6.5F—US shows a poorly defined, mildly hypoechoic area thought to correspond to the enhancing area on MRI.
- Figure 6.5G—Demonstrates an incidental small papilloma in an ectatic retroareolar duct on the contralateral breast.
- Figures 6.5H–I—Digital mammographic films after localization and bracketing of abnormal MRI enhancement, demonstrating postbiopsy changes and two metallic clips (one from targeted US biopsy and one from MRI core biopsy).

WORKUP

- Targeted US was performed and demonstrated a vague hypoechoic area corresponding in location to the suspicious MRI finding. US core biopsy was performed, which demonstrated sclerosing adenosis. This was considered discordant with the MRI findings and therefore MRI core biopsy was recommended. MRI-guided core biopsy was performed and demonstrated the presence of papilloma. In view of her high-risk status and suspicious nature of MRI findings, the area was bracketed and excised. Surgical excisional biopsy demonstrated papillomatosis and complex sclerosing lesion/radial scar.

DISCUSSION

For radial scars, MRI findings demonstrate distortion and spiculation, which may or may not enhance. We present this case because these findings can mimic breast carcinomas when they enhance. A spiculated mammographic lesion also may represent a malignancy or radial scar. If MRI is requested to evaluate this type of mammographic lesion, do *not* use absence of enhancement as a reason to defer biopsy. We recommend excision when radial scar is seen on core biopsy. Although a benign lesion, we have seen several cases in which excision of a radial scar has yielded an adjacent area of ductal carcinoma in situ.

• CASE 6

HISTORY

A 53-year-old woman with a positive family history of breast cancer presenting for high-risk screening MRI. Her mammogram demonstrated heterogeneously dense breasts without focal finding; bilateral screening sonography was also negative. MRI demonstrated a slightly irregular linear enhancing foci in the left central breast.

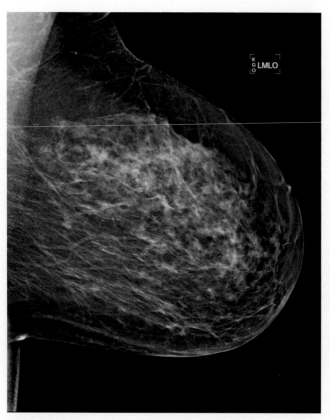

Figure 6.6A

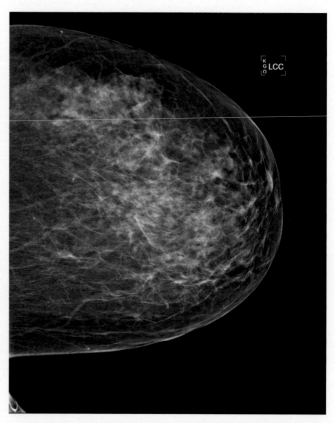

Figure 6.6B

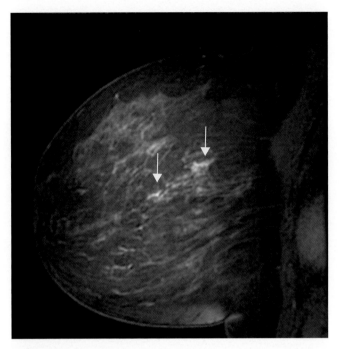

Figure 6.6C

FINDINGS

- Figures 6.6A–B—Digital mammogram images with heterogeneously dense parenchyma and no abnormality.
- Figure 6.6C—Postcontrast sagittal image at the time of core biopsy demonstrating irregular linear enhancing foci.

WORKUP

- MRI-guided core biopsy was performed and demonstrated LCIS. Localization and excision of the biopsy site was performed and demonstrated LCIS with a 1-mm focus of microinvasive lobular carcinoma.

DISCUSSION

LCIS has a varied appearance on MRI. A linear area of enhancement (similar to DCIS) is a common presentation. Classic teaching is that LCIS is an incidental finding on pathology with no associated finding on digital mammography. With MRI, this is not the case; LCIS can demonstrate findings that are confirmed by core, excisional biopsy, and postexcisional follow-up imaging. Other appearances we have seen that yield LCIS on biopsy include clumped enhancement or grouped enhancing foci.

• Plate 1

HISTORY

Another area of linear enhancement that was found to represent LCIS, in a different patient undergoing high-risk screening. This is a 55-year-old woman with strongly positive family history of breast cancer.

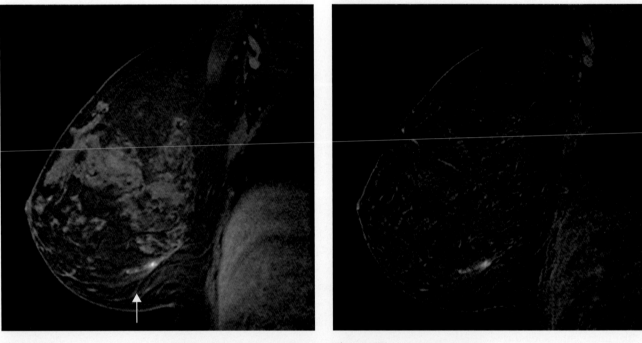

Plate 6.1A

Plate 6.1B

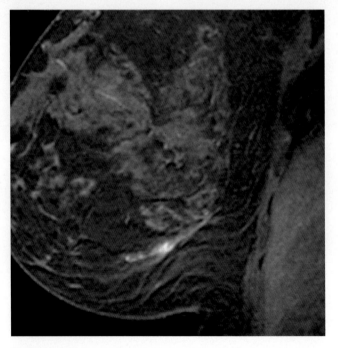

Plate 6.1C

FINDINGS

- Plate 6.1A—Post contrast.
- Plate 6.1B—Subtraction.
- Plate 6.1C—Magnified post-contrast, all demonstrating an area of linear "ductal appearing" enhancement.
- Again, core excisional biopsy yielded LCIS, with no residual suspicious enhancement remaining on postsurgical follow-up MRI scans.

• Plate 2

HISTORY

This is a third woman who had a history of DCIS found as an area of linear enhancement in the right breast. She was treated with lumpectomy and a bilateral reduction mammoplasty. In the contralateral (left) breast, a small area of linear enhancement was noted and thought to be suspicious for contralateral DCIS, but demonstrated LCIS on core biopsy and subsequent excision. Note the similiar appearances in DCIS and LCIS in this patient.

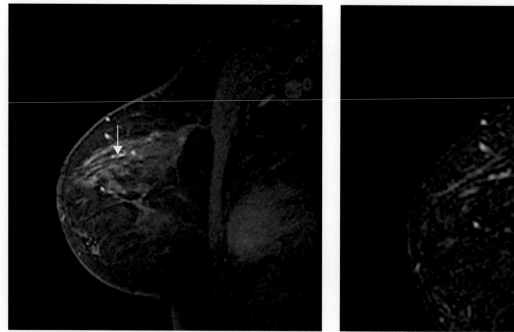

Plate 6.2A

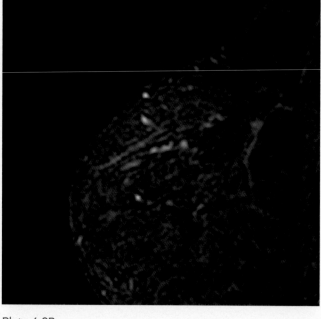

Plate 6.2B

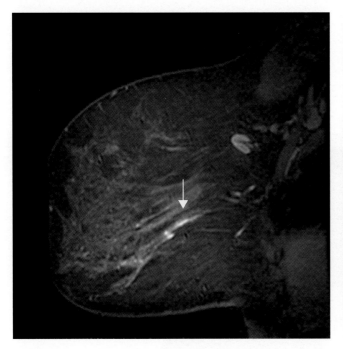

Plate 6.2C

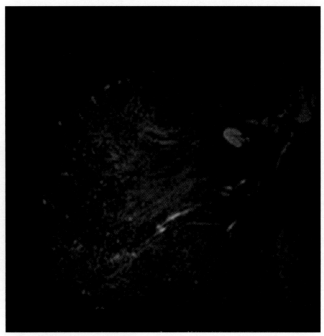

Plate 6.2D

FINDINGS

- Plates 6.2A–B—Post contrast & magnified subtraction images of the post-reduction LEFT breast, demonstrating a linear enhancing focus (arrow).

- Plates 6.2C–D—Post contrast & subtraction images of the RIGHT breast, prior to surgery. A larger area of linear enhancement is seen.

- Postcontrast subtracted and magnified images of left breast demonstrate linear enhancement in a "dot-dash" appearance, found to represent LCIS. This appearance can also be seen with DCIS.

- Figures P6.2C–D show the area of intense linear enhancement/DCIS in the right breast on postcontrast and subtracted images.

• Plate 3

HISTORY

An example of atypical hyperplasia found in a 50-year-old woman undergoing high-risk annual screening.

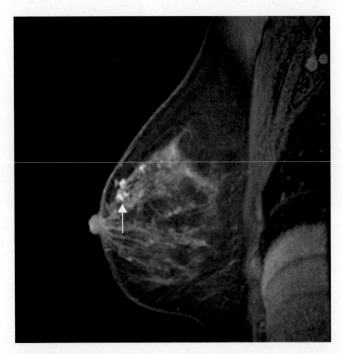

Plate 6.3

DISCUSSION

Nodular clumped enhancement is seen in the supraareolar region (see arrow Plate 6.3). The majority of MRI lesions demonstrating atypia do not have highly suspicious findings. The more typical findings on MRI for high-risk lesions is nodular or clumped non-masslike enhancement, usually without spiculation or distortion. Nodular clumped enhancement can also be very nonspecific and can be associated with benign non–high-risk lesions (e.g., hyperplasia/fibrocystic changes). The MRI appearance of atypia can overlap with benign glandular enhancement. Most of the lesions that we see that are high risk tend to demonstrate progressive or plateau enhancement kinetics. Occasionally they can demonstrate more suspicious washout kinetics. We have found that enhancement kinetics has not been helpful in distinguishing high-risk lesions from other benign lesions.

• CASE 1

HISTORY

A 59-year-old woman who presented with an abnormal screening mammogram demonstrating a cluster of heterogeneous calcifications in the left outer breast.

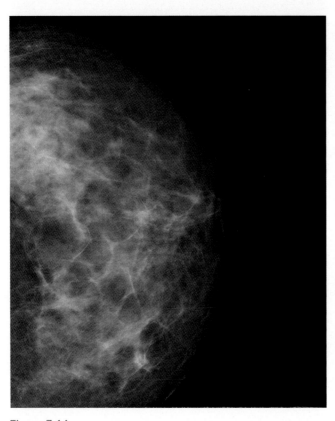

Figure 7.1A

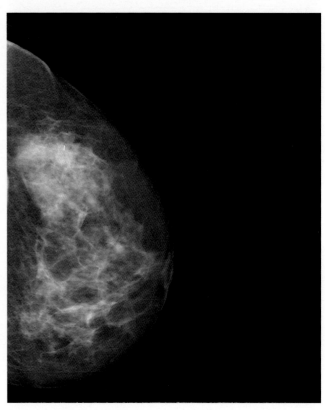

Figure 7.1B

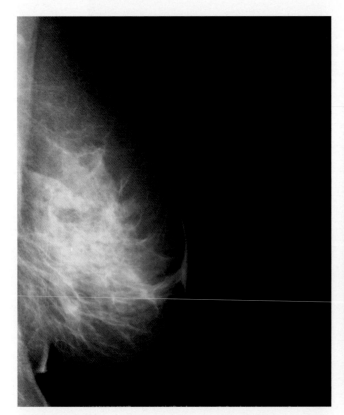

Figure 7.1C

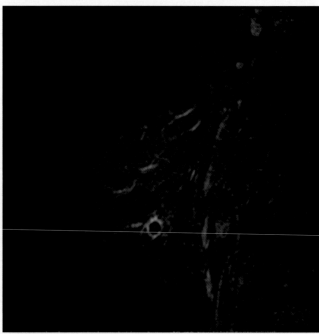

Figure 7.1D

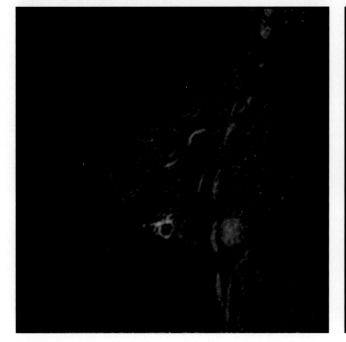

Figure 7.1E

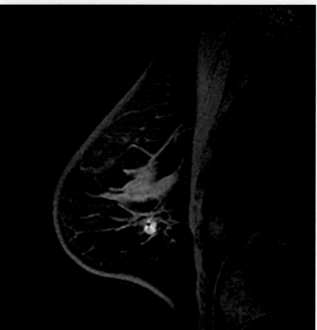

Figure 7.1F

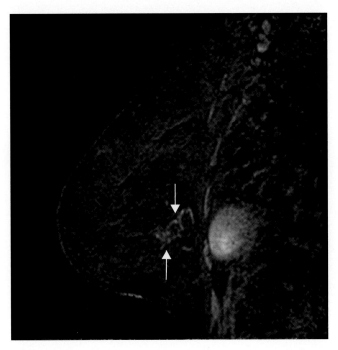

Figure 7.1G

FINDINGS

- Figure 7.1A—Demonstrating a small cluster of calcifications (laterally) and dense breasts.
- Figures 7.1B–C—Demonstrates post biopsy clip placement in the 3 to 4:00 axis in the left breast. The cluster was completely removed. The core biopsy demonstrated ductal carcinoma in situ (DCIS).
- Figures 7.1D–E—Magnetic resonance imaging (MRI) subtraction images of the biopsy cavity. In addition to the thin rim of enhancement usually seen around a biopsy site, there are some radiating enhancing spicules suggestive of residual neoplasm.
- Figure 7.1F—Demonstrates biopsy cavity with a high signal from blood (precontrast image & clip).
- Figure 7.1G—Demonstrates a central to inner near area, but not contiguous with, the suspicious area, which shows a segment of reticular nodular ('dot-dash') enhancement, extending over 3cm, suspicious for additional area of DCIS.

WORKUP

- MRI was done for extent of disease evaluation. On MRI, the cavity was noted with surrounding nodules/spiculated enhancement, suggesting residual malignancy, as well as the additional area of enhancement medial to the biopsy cavity. The patient refused needle-guided biopsy of this second area, electing to expedite the surgery. This area was thought to possibly be close enough in proximity to the original lesion, and the breast large enough to allow for cosmesis, to enable bracketing of the area at the time of the lumpectomy.

DISCUSSION

In this case, core biopsy was not attempted at the second site because of patient refusal. However, you must recommend sampling any additional areas with needle core biopsy *before* surgical intervention, because this may affect surgical planning and decision. The final pathology after bracketing the area on MRI demonstrated extensive DCIS (>7 cm involvement) from 3 to 6:00 axis of the left breast. She ultimately required a mastectomy.

This type of appearance of DCIS can be easily overlooked or confused with background enhancement. It is often progressive and best visualized on the delayed series (fourth post-contrast series) as opposed to the first. Subtraction images aid greatly in seeing subtle signs of DCIS because the surrounding structures become less conspicuous.

With compression for procedures, this subtle type of enhancement may be delayed or even obliterated. If you are strongly suspicious of a lesion, but not seeing enhancement at the time of planned MRI-guided core biopsy, consider sampling the area anyway via landmarks/location.

• CASE 2

HISTORY

A 77-year-old woman presents with an abnormal outside screening mammogram read as Breast Imaging-Reporting and Data System (BIRADS) 0/incomplete demonstrating clustered calcifications in the 6:00 to 7:00 axis of the right breast, questionably vascular, loosely grouped. Breast MRI was recommended for further evaluation.

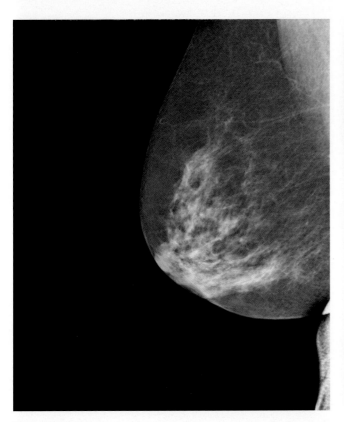

Figure 7.2A

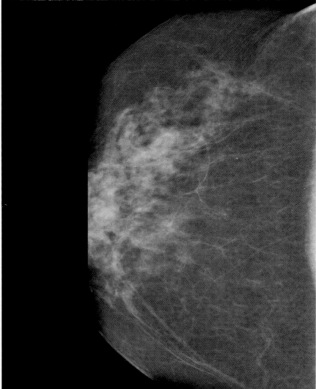

Figure 7.2B

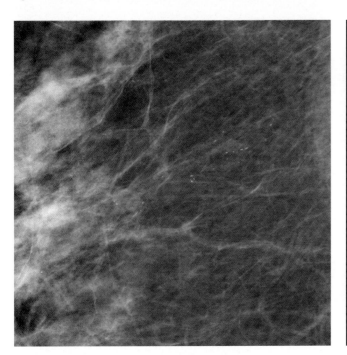

Figure 7.2C

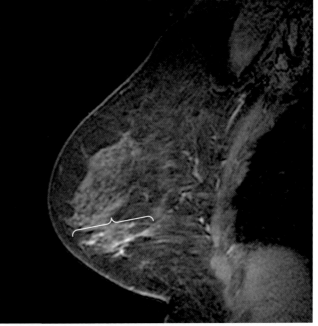

Figure 7.2D

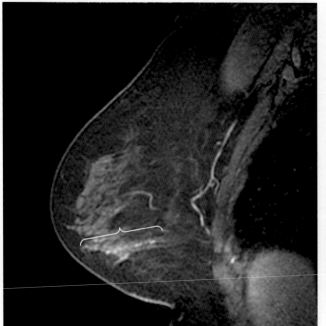

Figure 7.2E

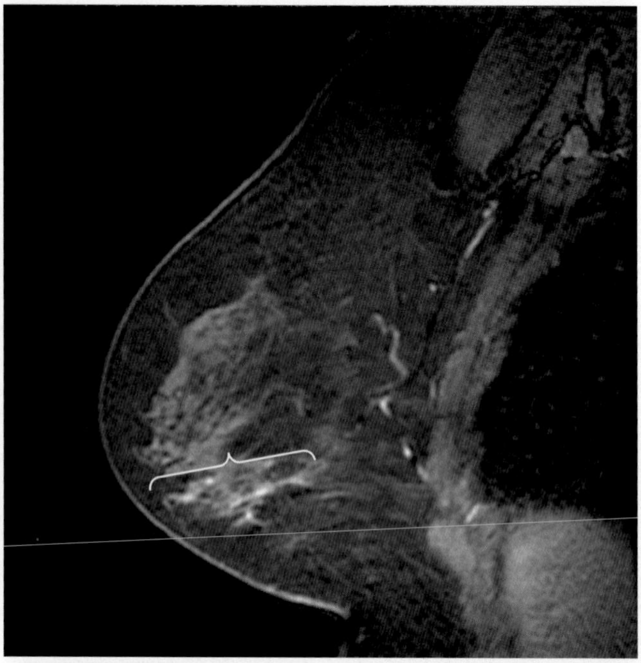

Figure 7.2F

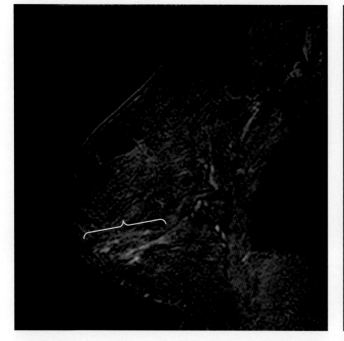

Figure 7.2G

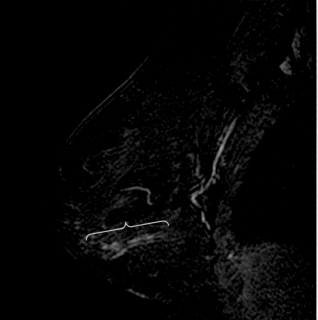

Figure 7.2H

FINDINGS

- Figures 7.2A–C—Digital mammography including magnification views performed at follow-up demonstrating mixed fibroglandular tissue with heterogeneous clustered ductal appearing calcifications in the 6:00 to 7:00 axis in a segmental distribution.
- Figures 7.2D–F—Demonstrates postcontrast images of the same region.
- Figures 7.2G–H—Subtracted images demonstrating linear enhancing foci in a segmental distribution with a dot-dash appearance. Note that the findings became more conspicuous when viewed on the subtracted images. It is still visible without the subtraction, but because it is a relatively subtle finding, can be overlooked or mistaken for glandular enhancement on the nonsubtracted image.

WORKUP

- The initial MRI was read as probable glandular enhancement and a 6-month follow-up was recommended. The outside mammogram images were not available at the time of initial MRI interpretation. On 6-month follow-up, digital mammography demonstrated a relatively large area of heterogeneous calcifications, some of which were linear/ductal in morphology. MRI demonstrated a large segmental region of reticular nodular ("dot/dash") enhancement radiating toward the nipple with small nodular enhancing foci. A stereotactic core biopsy was performed; pathology demonstrated ductal carcinoma in situ. The area was bracketed for excision. Final pathology demonstrated 2-mm invasive ductal carcinoma with surrounding extensive DCIS.

DISCUSSION

Several points are illustrated in this case. The most important point is to always review the mammograms and breast ultrasounds before making final recommendations on MRI exams, because they can markedly influence your reading. In addition, as the one who interprets the MRI, your recommendation is frequently considered to supersede (sometimes erroneously!) any previous mammogram/sonogram report. When indeterminate calcifications are visualized on digital mammography, MRI should *not* be ordered to resolve them. Stereotactic biopsy should have been performed. MRI was inappropriately requested to evaluate calcifications, and the mistake was somewhat compounded by overlooking the subtle appearance of DCIS on MRI. When the patient returned 6 months later and the findings were more prominent, the diagnosis was easily made and appropriate treatment ensued.

We have had many cases in which the index lesion on mammogram was small, but the suspicious region of enhancement is relatively large on MRI. Whenever possible, we bracket the area for excision using as guidance the imaging modality on which the lesion is largest. We recommend bracketing for most lesions lager than 2.5 to 3 cm, depending on the breast size. A small-breasted woman cannot have a large carcinoma resected for breast conservation therapy and still have an acceptable cosmetic result. If breast size is of concern, or the area is felt to be possibly too large for breast conservation, a second core biopsy of the farthest away suspicious site should be considered before final surgical planning. Even with bracketing, it still will not ensure negative margins (although it helps guide surgeon) because microscopic foci cannot be visualized with any imaging modality. The details of surgical planning should be done in conjunction with the surgeon.

• CASE 3

HISTORY

A 29-year-old woman with a strong family history for breast cancer presented with a palpable mass in the right outer breast, but negative digital mammography and sonography.

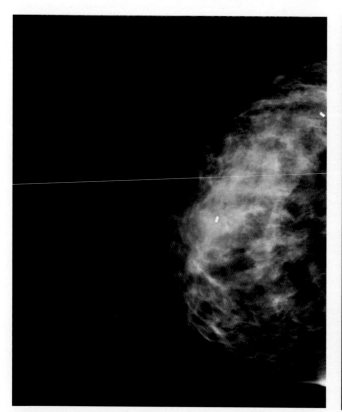

Figure 7.3A

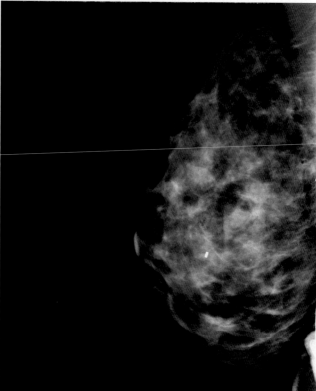

Figure 7.3B

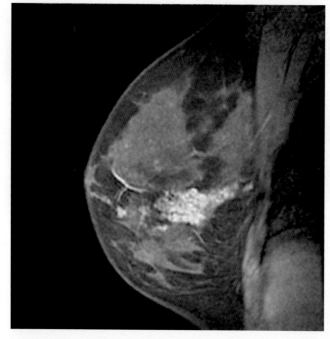

Figure 7.3C

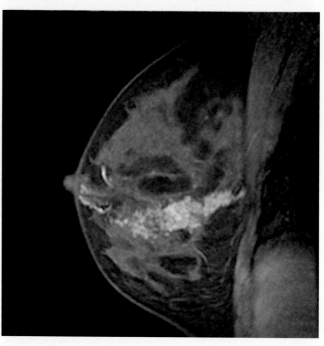

Figure 7.3D

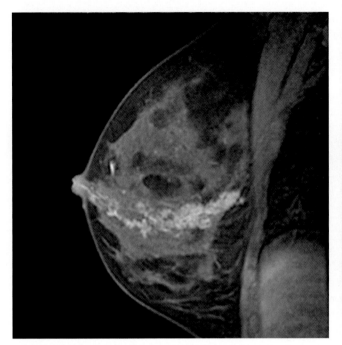

Figure 7.3E

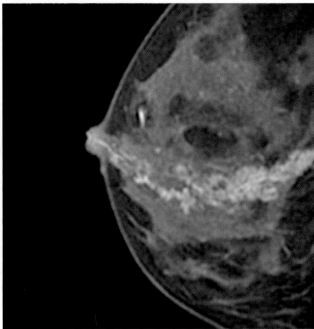

Figure 7.3F

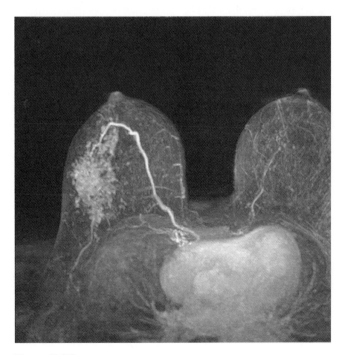

Figure 7.3G

FINDINGS

- Figures 7.3A–B—Demonstrate the postbiopsy digital mammography with two clips, approximately 8 cm apart, on a background of heterogeneously dense parenchyma. No calcifications are seen.

- Figures 7.3C–E—Clumped linear, and nodular enhancement in a segmental distribution, radiating from or toward the nipple, a pattern that is highly suspicious for DCIS. With this volume of abnormal enhancement, an invasive component is not unexpected.

- Figure 7.3F—Magnified view showing enhancement extending into the nipple.

- Figure 7.3G—Three-dimensional computer aided diagnosis (CAD) image demonstrating the anatomical extent of the lesion.

WORK-UP

- An MRI was performed for clinical problem solving. In the area of the palpable abnormality, there is a large segmental area of clumped and linear enhancement, extending from the posterior aspect of the breast into the nipple. This is a highly suspicious for malignancy and biopsy was recommended. Anterior and posterior areas were targeted to help preoperative planning, for decision regarding attempted lumpectomy versus mastectomy. Both areas were found to contain DCIS on core biopsy. She underwent mastectomy, which demonstrated 10 cm of DCIS, intermediate grade, no invasive disease, and no lymph node metastases.

DISCUSSION

A woman who presents with a palpable mass, but negative mammogram and breast ultrasound, should be considered for MRI for clinical problem solving. Although intermediate palpable masses will be removed by the surgeon anyway, knowing the true nature of the mass prior to surgery enables appropriate surgical planning. After needle confirmation of diagnosis, appropriate treatment (lumpectomy vs. mastectomy), and appropriate lymph node sampling (sentinel node vs. axillary dissection) can be selected. Remember that no matter how suspicious the lesion is on MRI, pathologic confirmation (via needle biopsy) is necessary before treatment. In addition, a decision to proceed with mastectomy as opposed to breast conservation should also be made with preoperative pathologic proof that extent of disease warrants that surgery (e.g., >5 cm lesion, more than one quadrant of involvement). This patient had an initial core biopsy performed in the clinician's office with benign pathology. Because of suspicious clinical findings, MRI was requested. The true extent of the disease was not apparent clinically, but is obvious on MRI. In addition, the better visualization allowed more optimal targeting for core biopsies than would have been possible without imaging.

Nowadays many women with breast cancer, especially younger ones, are electing bilateral mastectomy for their treatment of choice. Although this may shorten the workup, it should never be chosen for that purpose. Additional biopsies should be performed as quickly, as comfortably, and as least stressfully as possible for the patient. Even if a patient is electing mastectomy, it is wise to sample additional suspicious lesions before surgery. This way, if no synchronous lesion is noted in mastectomy specimen, the patient will not second guess herself (or her physician) and regret her decision to undergo mastectomy.

Our nurse navigator will inform every newly diagnosed breast cancer patient that additional areas of "sampling" will frequently and routinely take place, and that we do this so that the surgical treatment can be customized for their particular case, and to help ensure that only one visit to the operating room will be necessary.

The radiologist should be aware that even when biopsy proven synchronous disease is present, the pathologist can easily overlook this when examining the mastectomy specimen. Unless otherwise informed, they evaluate the main tumor and take only random sections from the remaining three quadrants of the breast. Clip placement will greatly enhance your radiologic/pathologic correlation.

We do not use our three-dimensional imaging much during interpretation, but this is a very useful tool to demonstrate the suspected volume of tumor relative to breast size for the clinicians/surgeons (and patients, when appropriate). Although this 29-year-old patient had a strongly positive family history, she had not begun high-risk screening. The American Cancer Society suggests that women who are at risk begin screening earlier (ages 30–35, or 5–10 years before the age that their family members were diagnosed).

• **CASE 4**

HISTORY

A 47-year-old woman who presented with calcifications in the left inner upper quadrant on screening digital mammography. Stereotactic biopsy demonstrated DCIS.

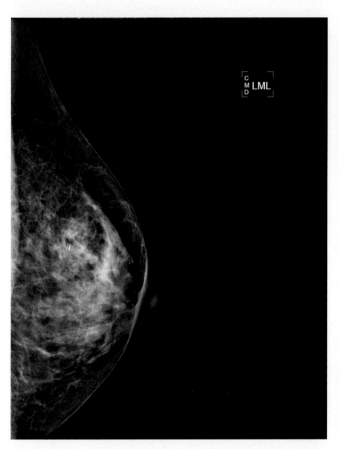

Figure 7.4A

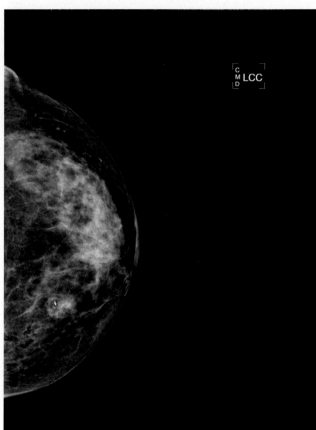

Figure 7.4B

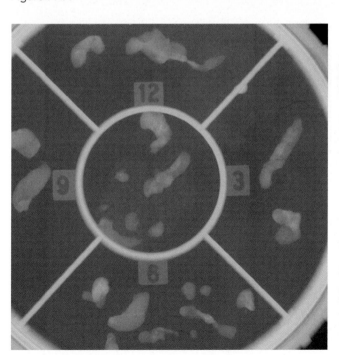

Figure 7.4C

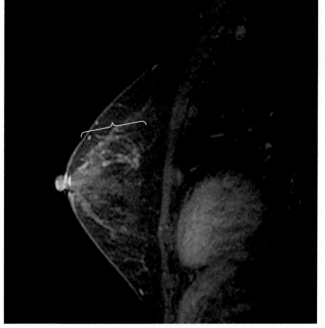

Figure 7.4D

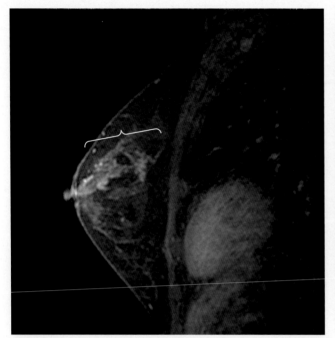

Figure 7.4E

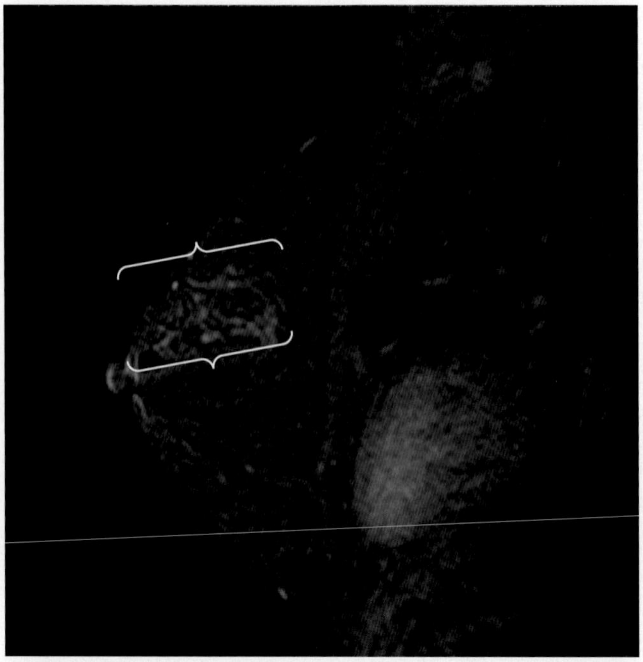

Figure 7.4F

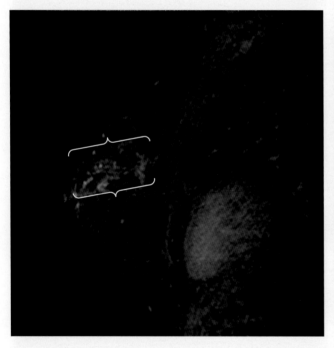

Figure 7.4G

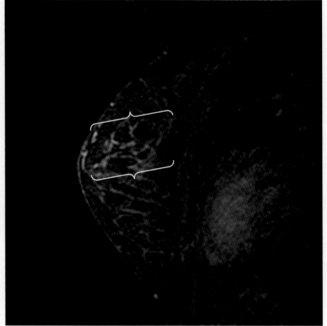

Figure 7.4H

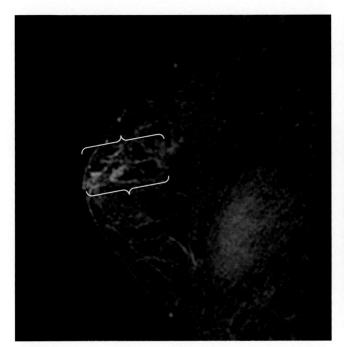

Figure 7.4I

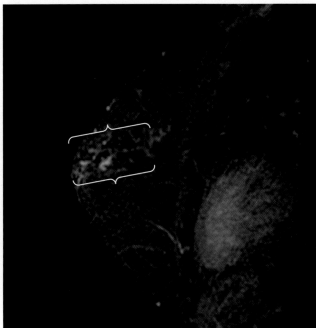

Figure 7.4J

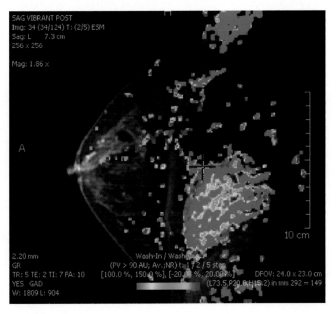

Figure 7.4K

FINDINGS

- Figures 7.4A–B—Postbiopsy mammogram demonstrating heterogeneously dense mammogram and clip in the area of concern. No residual calcifications are seen on standard views.

- Figure 7.4C—Digital magnification views of cores, showing all the calcifications have been excised.

- Figures 7.4D–E—Postcontrast demonstrates small enhancing foci scattered in the left upper inner quadrant.

- Figure 7.4F—The early subtraction images demonstrate the reticular nodular pattern of enhancement, which is subtle but visible. Always be suspicious of this appearance, especially in the setting of evaluation for extent of disease/DCIS. The subtraction of the background makes subtle abnormalities more visible.

- Figure 7.4G–J—The delayed subtraction images makes the enhancement (because it is predominantly progressive) more prominent. Now the areas of enhancement are larger and some have the appearance of clumped enhancement.

- Figure 7.4K—Color enhanced kinetic analysis (computer aided diagnosis/CAD) image demonstrates low level predominantly progressive enhancement.

WORKUP

- Calcifications were completely removed on core biopsy as confirmed by postbiopsy mammogram. Prior to surgery she had an extent of disease work up with MRI. MRI demonstrated extremely subtle reticular nodular enhancement throughout the left upper inner quadrant with a minimal amount of clumped enhancement in the retroareolar region. She was found to have extensive DCIS at time of lumpectomy, and eventually required mastectomy. Final pathology demonstrated extensive DCIS, no invasion, and negative lymph nodes.

DISCUSSION

On the first postcontrast scans, DCIS may be overlooked on MRI because it tends to exhibit more delayed (progressive or plateau) enhancement, as compared with invasive neoplasms which are more frequently associated with early rapid enhancement and washout. Also, because of the subtle nature of some of these lesions, the radiologist may fail to recognize them. In the literature, low-grade DCIS is believed to be less detectable on MRI than high-grade DCIS. In our experience, we have not found this to always be the case; rather, we have noted the size of the lesion is much more closely correlated with visibility than the grade of the lesion. The presence or absence of background glandular enhancement also closely influences the visibility of areas of DCIS.

• CASE 5

HISTORY

A 36-year-old woman who presented with an abnormal baseline screening mammogram with numerous calcifications throughout the right breast.

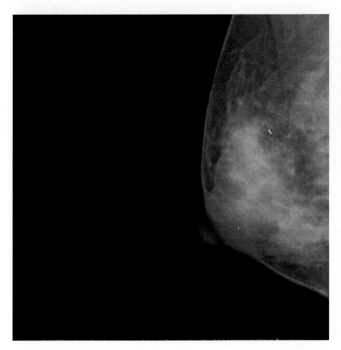

Figure 7.5A

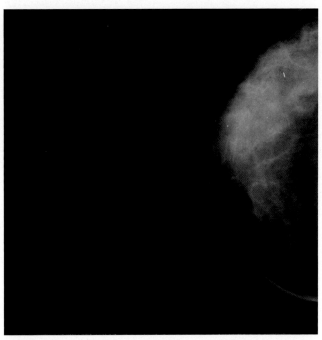

Figure 7.5B

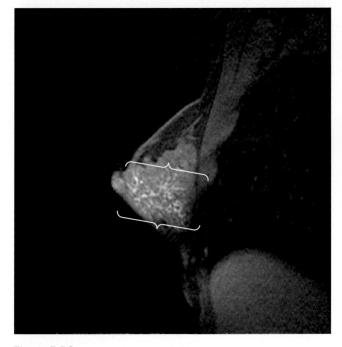

Figure 7.5C

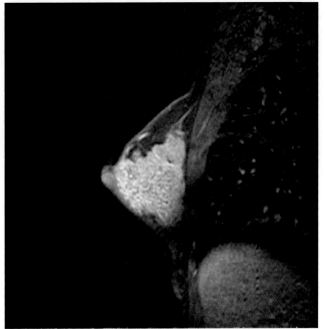

Figure 7.5D

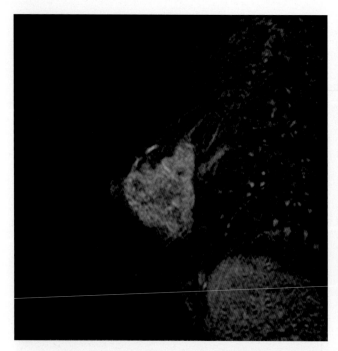

Figure 7.5E

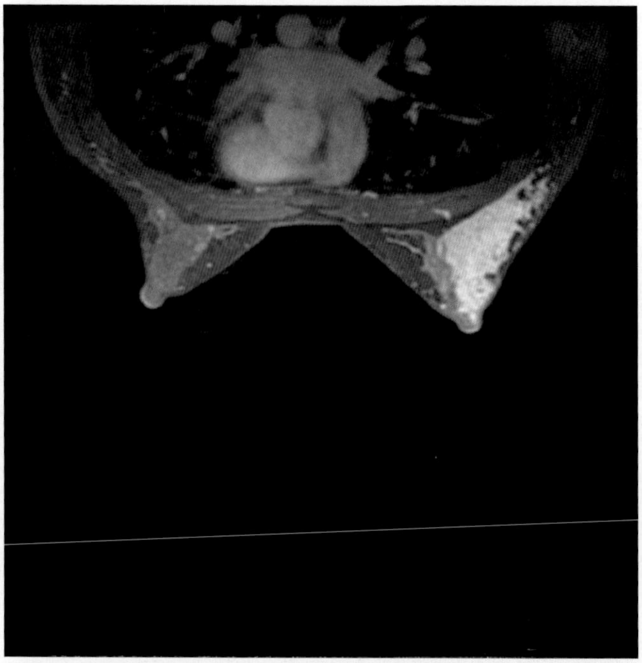

Figure 7.5F

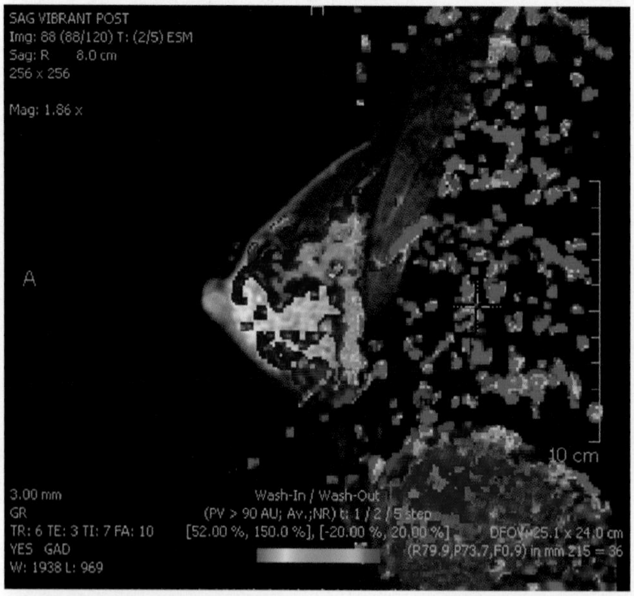

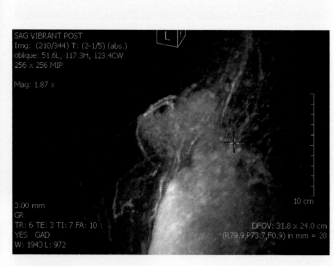

Figure 7.5G

Figure 7.5H

FINDINGS

- Figures 7.5A–B—Mammogram demonstrating diffuse calcifications in three quadrants with dense parenchyma. Because of the diffuse calcifications, the differential diagnosis included sclerosing adenosis/fibrocystic changes as well as malignancy.

- Figure 7.5C—MRI, first postcontrast series demonstrating reticular nodular enhancement throughout the breast.

- Figure 7.5D—Fourth postcontrast series. The enhancement coalesces and appears more solid and diffuse.

- Figure 7.5E—Subtracted contrast series. Again, the diffuse enhancement in the entire outer breast (upper and lower) is seen.

- Figure 7.5F—Delayed axial images. The outer two thirds of the right breast enhances intensely.

- Figure 7.5G—Color analysis CAD image demonstrates very heterogeneous kinetics, but predominantly of the progressive and plateau type. Again, washout is not always seen in malignant lesions. Marked heterogeneity of enhancement types does seem to be more common in cancers, and homogeneity of enhancement kinetics seems to be more common in benign lesions.

- Figure 7.5H—3-dimensional CAD image gives an impressive overview of the volume of breast tissue involved with DCIS in this patient. This is a useful tool to display involved areas to clinicians. Clinicians are less able to translate pathology visualized only on sagittal and axial sections into a three-dimensional picture of the actual tumor burden. While a radiologist may rarely need the 3D reconstruction to understand the extent of disease clinicians are very appriciation of this feature.

WORKUP

- Stereotactic biopsy was performed and demonstrated the presence of DCIS. MRI was performed for extent of disease. Two thirds of the breast demonstrated abnormal enhancement. She was then brought back for additional stereotactic biopsies. Two additional quadrants were sampled and also demonstrated DCIS. She underwent mastectomy. Final pathology—extensive DCIS (>8 cm) with 1 positive sentinel node. No invasion could be found on resectioning of the specimen however; presumably a focus (or foci) of microinvasion must be present, because lymph node involvement was discovered.

DISCUSSION

When an abnormality is this large, it can be difficult to diagnose on imaging because there is no normal surrounding tissue to make the abnormality more conspicuous. In this case, the abnormality is most visible on the axial delayed images, because we have the comparison of the normal contralateral breast. Sometimes the MRI can be used to plan additional biopsies of other suspicious areas on mammogram or ultrasound. The geographic appearance of the DCIS in this case is striking and unusual.

As an aside, we have seen geographic patterns of enhancement similar to this appearance in lactating breasts (Fig. 7.5F).

• CASE 6

HISTORY

A 46-year-old woman who presented with an abnormal screening mammogram, which demonstrated an asymmetric density in the right inner breast seen on the cc view only.

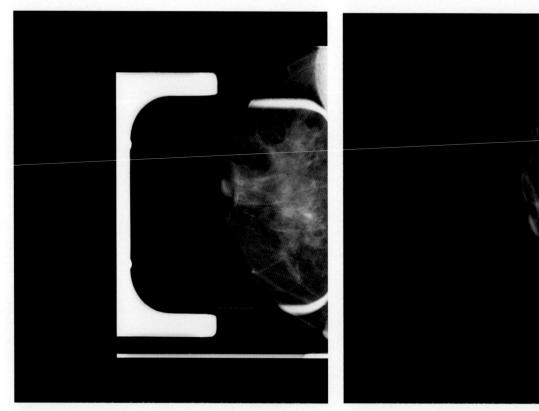

Figure 7.6A   Figure 7.6B

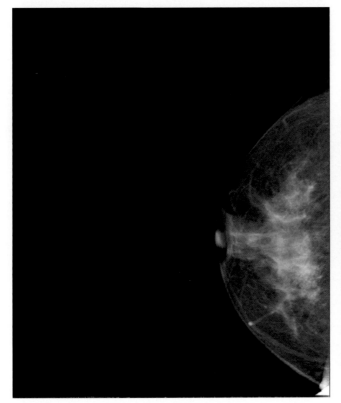

Figure 7.6C

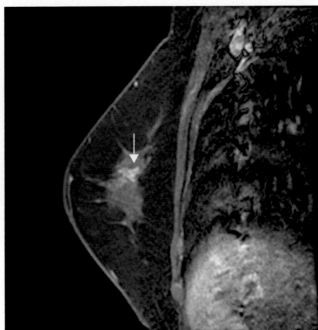

Figure 7.6D

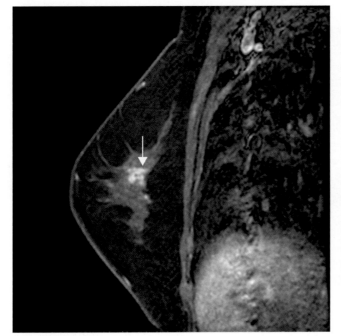

Figure 7.6E

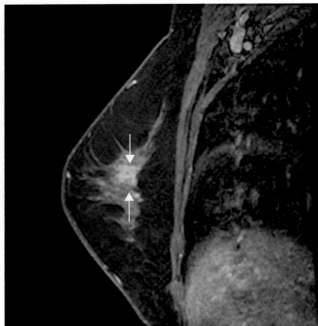

Figure 7.6F

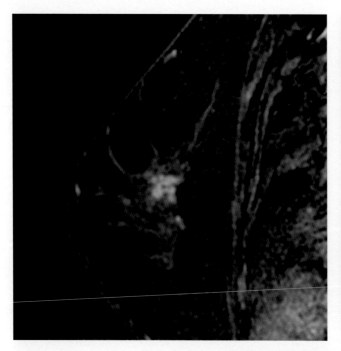

Figure 7.6G

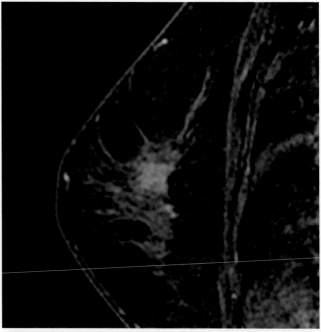

Figure 7.6H

FINDINGS

- Figures 7.6A–C—spot compression, MLO, and CC views from digital mammography demonstrating a vague area of asymmetric density (with one or two calcifications) which appeared more prominent than on prior exams.
- Figures 7.6D–E—Demonstrates first postcontrast series with irregular, clumped, and nodular enhancement with some grouped enhancing foci. This area had mixed enhancing kinetics including areas of washout.
- Figure 7.6F—Demonstrates fourth postcontrast series, showing washout as well as the "blossoming" effect in which the margins appear to spread out.
- Figure 7.6G—Subtracted first postcontrast series.
- Figure 7.6H—Subtracted fourth postcontrast series.

WORKUP

- Additional spot views and ultrasound demonstrated a vague area of soft tissue density with occasional calcifications in the inner breast, but no discrete corresponding finding on the lateral view or on ultrasound. MRI was recommended for mammographic problem solving. MRI demonstrated an area of clumped irregular enhancement with some washout enhancement kinetics in the right inner breast 9:00 axis, which corresponded to the area of concern on mammogram. MRI core biopsy was performed and demonstrated DCIS. She underwent lumpectomy, which demonstrated a 1.2-cm high-grade DCIS.

DISCUSSION

Notice the appearance of the area on the fourth postcontrast series compared with the first postcontrast series. This is due to a number of factors. By the fourth series, the background normal tissue begins to enhance slowly, so we lose the pictoral contrast between the lesion and the background. In addition, areas of the tumor that are exhibiting washout kinetics are losing their contrast uptake. Third, the margins appear slightly expanded as if the area has "blossomed." This is even more obvious with areas of linear enhancement as the "line" appears to get thicker. This is probably related to the infiltrative margins of these neoplastic lesions, as opposed to benign lesions, which tend to have more sharply defined encapsulated margins. This is often best demonstrated on the subtracted series, as with any subtle finding on MRI.

• **Plate 1**

HISTORY

A 49-year-old woman, with high-risk screening MRI performed for positive family history. She had history of prior benign left breast core biopsies and negative bilateral mammography with heterogeneously dense breasts.

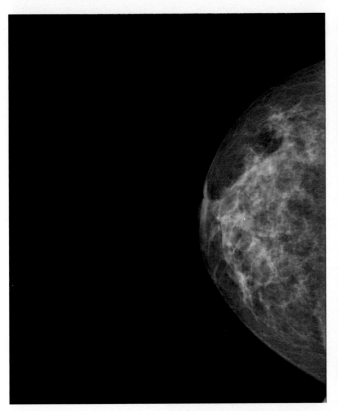

Plate 7.1A

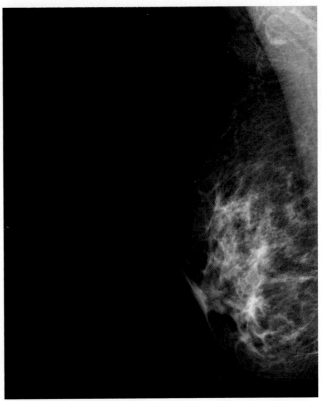

Plate 7.1B

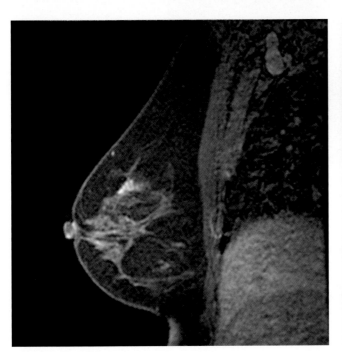

Plate 7.1C

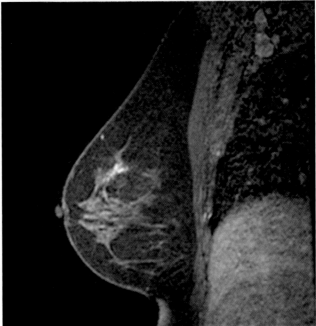

Plate 7.1D

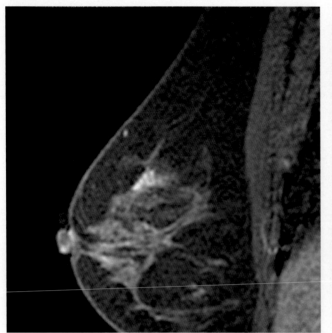

Plate 7.1E

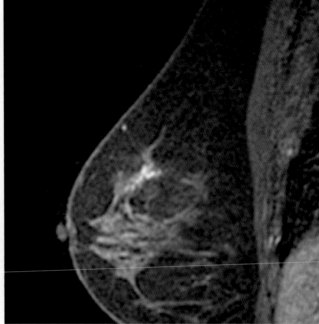

Plate 7.1F

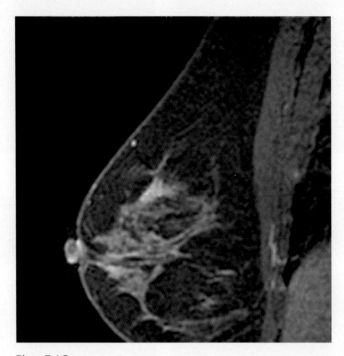

Plate 7.1G

FINDINGS

- Plates 7.1A–B—Demonstrated clip from core biopsy and heterogeneously dense parenchyma.
- Plates 7.1C–D—Demonstrating sagittal, postcontrast images with irregular linear and clumped enhancement in 12:00 axis of the right breast.
- Plates 7.1E–F—Magnified image of irregular enhancing area.
- Plate 7.1G—Fourth postcontrast series; the lesion appears to spread out. This reflects the indistinct margins of neoplastic involvement, as well as the "washout" of the contrast.

MRI core biopsy of this area was performed. It demonstrated presence of DCIS. She underwent lumpectomy with wire localization which revealed 0.8 cm of DCIS with microinvasion and surrounding microscopic foci of DCIS.

DISCUSSION

Any isolated area of clumped or linear enhancement could represent malignancy. If the margin is irregular, your level of suspicion should increase. On the other hand, clumped enhancement may also be associated with fibrocystic change or even glandular enhancement, so consider the morphology of margin features. Kinetic analysis may not be helpful in these cases, because DCIS and glandular enhancement may both exhibit progressive kinetics. Anecdotally, we have seen many cases of DCIS that appear larger in overall size on the last postcontrast sagittal series as compared to the first. This can be seen with invasive neoplasms as well, but this is less common in well circumscribed benign lesions (such as fibroadenomas, benign nodules, etc.). This probably reflects the encapsulated nature of many benign lesions, as compared with the infiltrative nature of the edge of most malignancies.

• **Plate 2**

HISTORY

A 46-year-old woman who presented with a one-view-only finding noted on mammogram that persisted on spot view, but could not be found on ultrasound. She has a history of a previous benign surgical biopsy.

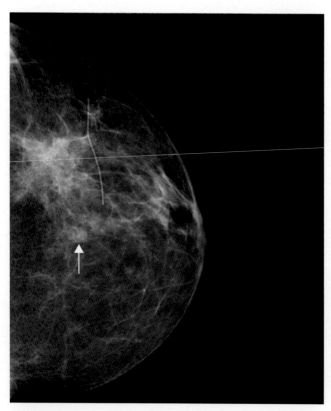

Plate 7.2A

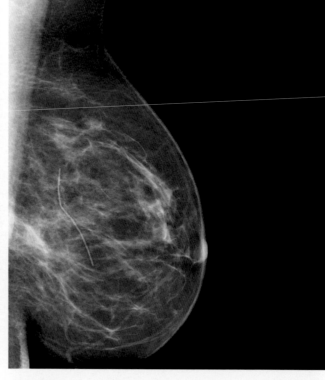

Plate 7.2B

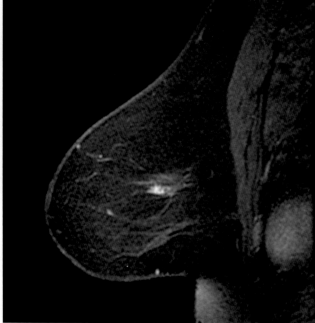

Plate 7.2C

Plate 7.2D

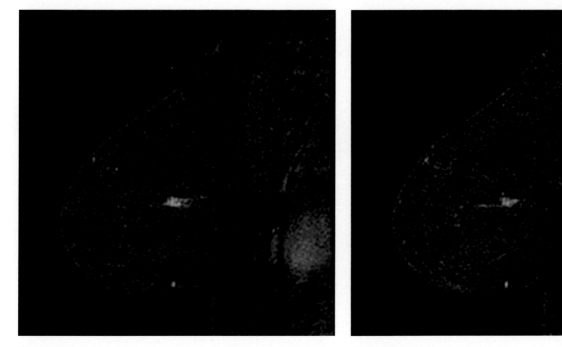

Plate 7.2E

Plate 7.2F

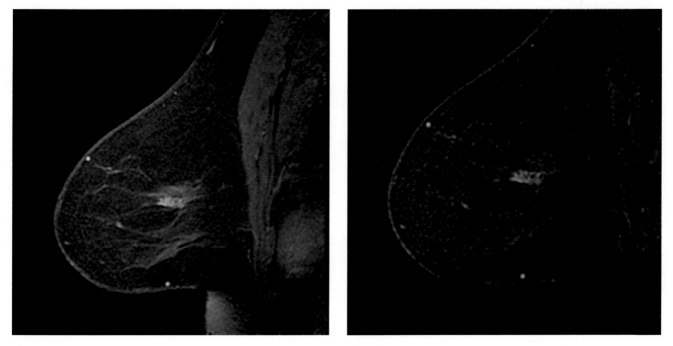

Plate 7.2G

Plate 7.2H

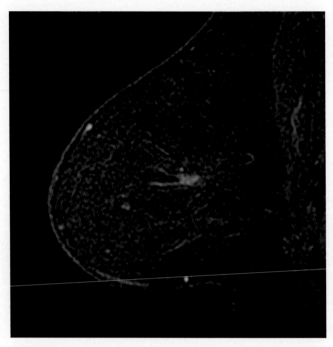

Plate 7.2I

FINDINGS

- Plates 7.2A–B—Demonstrate breast with mixed fibroglandular and fatty tissue with postsurgical changes in the outer lower quadrant and a 1.1 cm relatively smooth nodular density seen on the central breast (arrow).

- Plates 7.2C–D—First postcontrast series demonstrating an irregular area of clumped enhancement in the left central breast corresponding to the region of concern on digital mammography.

- Plates 7.2E–F—Subtracted images demonstrating obvious irregular clumped enhancement centrally, with an area of linear enhancement extending anteriorly toward the nipple, and to a lesser extent, posteriorly.

- Plates 7.2G–I—Fourth post contrast series demonstrating the "blossoming" effect of the lesion. The lesion appears to fill out and the linear enhancement is more visible on the subtracted series.

MRI core biopsy was performed, which demonstrated DCIS. Lumpectomy demonstrated 0.5-cm residual DCIS with atypical ductal hyperplasia.

• Plate 3

HISTORY

A 68-year-old woman with a family history of breast carcinoma, with negative routine screening mammogram and BIRADS 3 (probably benign) ultrasound for unrelated presumed complex cyst in the right breast.

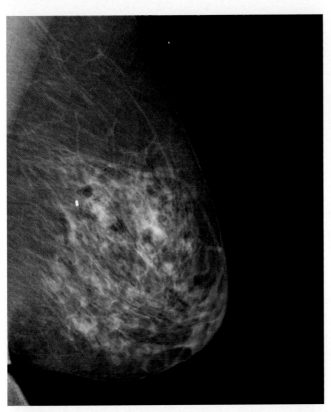

Plate 7.3A

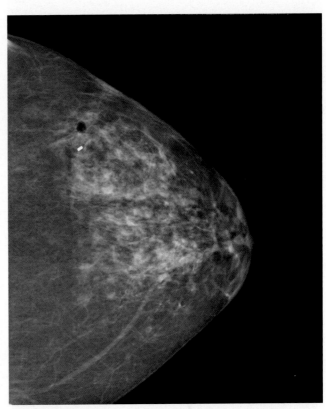

Plate 7.3B

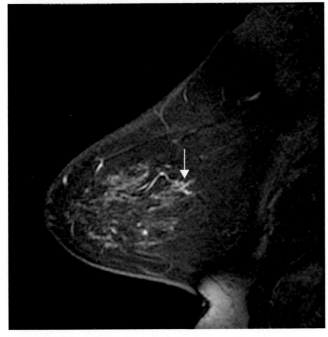

Plate 7.3C

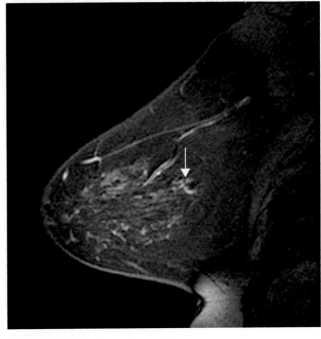

Plate 7.3D

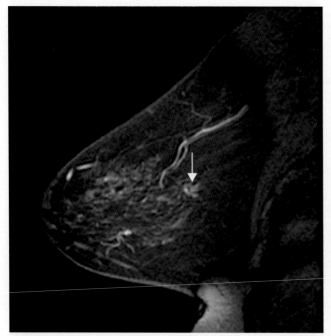

Plate 7.3E

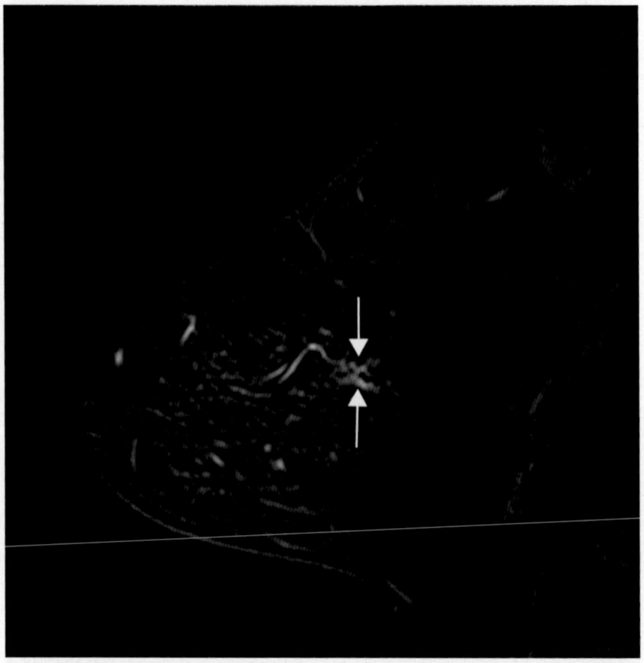

Plate 7.3F

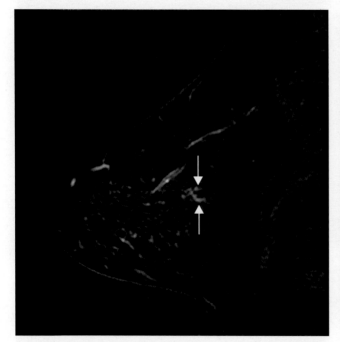

Plate 7.3G

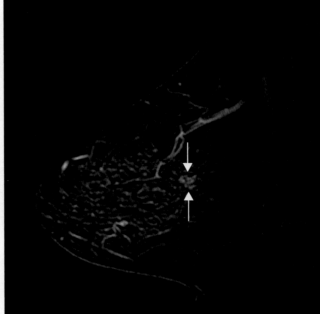

Plate 7.3H

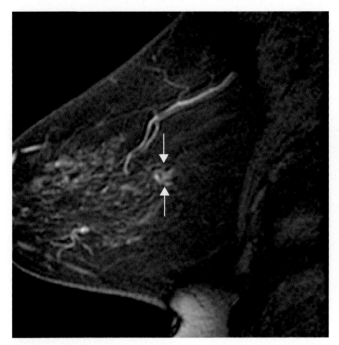

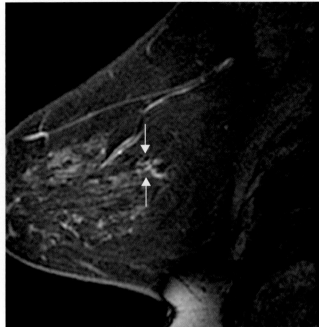

Plate 7.3I   Plate 7.3J

FINDINGS

- Plates 7.3A–B—Demonstrate heterogeneous dense parenchyma, post-MRI core with clip at biopsy site.

- Plates 7.3C–E—Demonstrating the first postcontrast series with linear and reticulonodular ("dot-dash") enhancement in the left upper outer quadrant.

- Plates 7.3F–G—Demonstrate the subtracted series, which make the lesion more conspicuous.

- Plate 7.3H—Demonstrates the fourth subtraction series.

- Plates 7.3I–J—Magnified contiguous sagittal postcontrast views demonstrating the enhancing area to be slightly spiculated, which raised the level of suspicion.

DISCUSSION

She had an MRI-guided core biopsy of the left upper outer quadrant area of enhancement that demonstrated DCIS. She underwent lumpectomy with wire localization, which demonstrated a 3.6-cm area of DCIS with multiple positive margins. This case demonstrates very minimal and subtle MRI findings for what proved to be a very large area of DCIS. Not all DCIS is visible on MRI. However, recognizing subtle findings will become easier as you have more experience interpreting breast MRI.

• Plate 4

HISTORY

A 66-year-old woman with an abnormal screening mammogram that demonstrated left breast 4:00 axis calcifications. Stereotactic core biopsy demonstrated DCIS. MRI was performed for extent of disease evaluation. She subsequently underwent lumpectomy with wire localization; final pathology demonstrated a 4.5-cm DCIS, comedo type, extending into a lactiferous duct at the nipple.

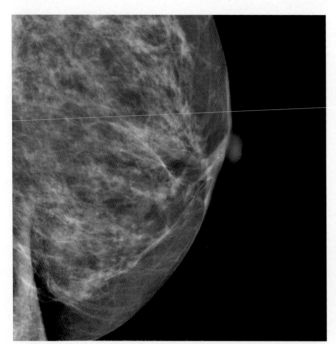

Plate 7.4A

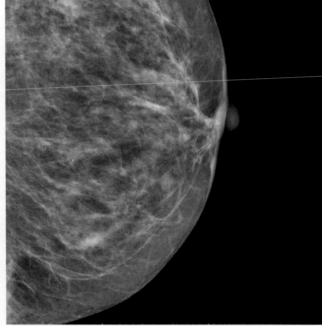

Plate 7.4B

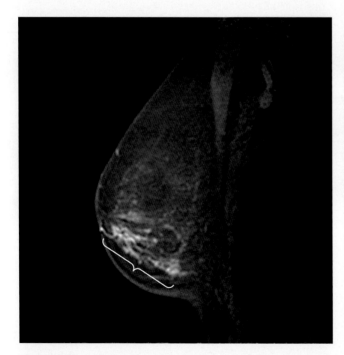

Plate 7.4C

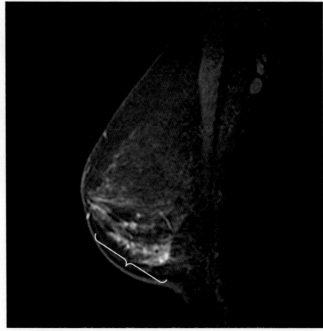

Plate 7.4D

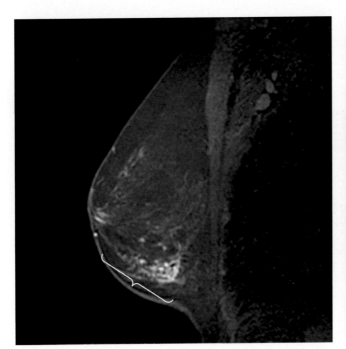

Plate 7.4E

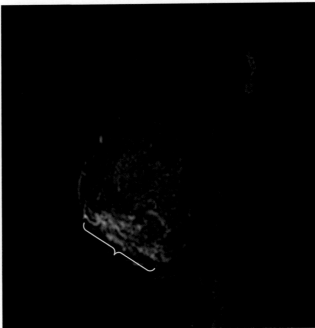

Plate 7.4F

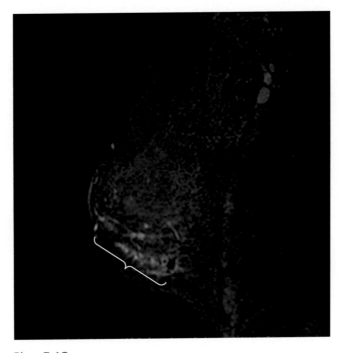

Plate 7.4G

FINDINGS

- Plates 7.4A–B—Magnified mammographic images demonstrating mixed fibroglandular/fatty tissue with pleomorphic casting type calcifications at the 4:00 axis, extending from the posterior third of the outer lower quadrant to the nipple.
- Plates 7.4C–D—Demonstrates postcontrast sagittal series with extensive segmentally distributed clumped nodular and linear enhancement extending from the left posterior outer lower quadrant to the nipple.
- Plates 7.4F–G—Subtracted series demonstrates similar findings.

DISCUSSION

In this particular case, the digital mammography and the MRI give virtually the same information as to the extent of the disease.

• Plate 5

HISTORY

A 57-year-old woman who presented for her high-risk screening MRI (positive family history of breast carcinoma), which demonstrated areas of enhancement in the right 10, 12, and 3:00. The most suspicious area is in the 3:00 axis. Routine screening mammogram had been negative. MRI-guided core biopsy was performed and demonstrated presence of DCIS at both the 3:00 and 12:00 axis. The 10:00 axis lesion was benign on core biopsy. She underwent mastectomy, which demonstrated Grade 2 cribriform DCIS at multiple sites.

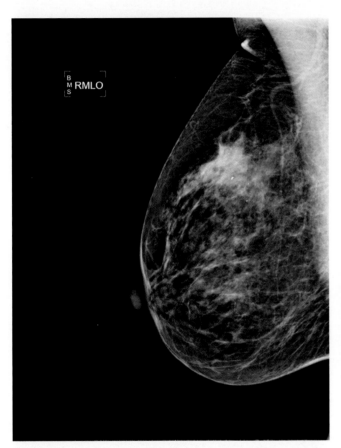

Plate 7.5A

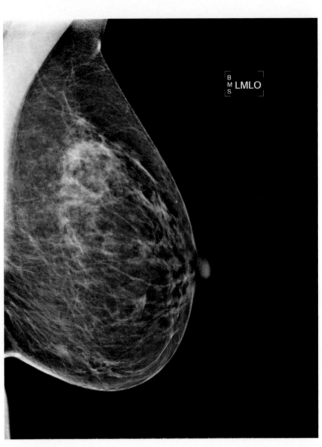

Plate 7.5B

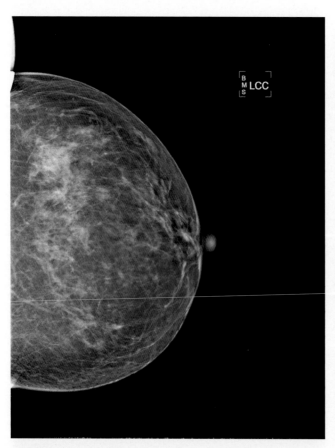

Plate 7.5C

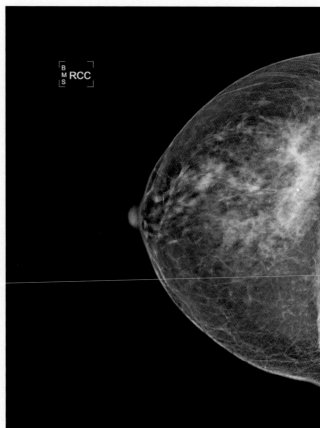

Plate 7.5D

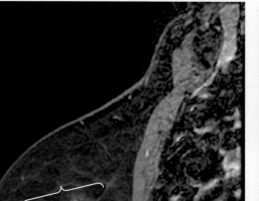

Plate 7.5E

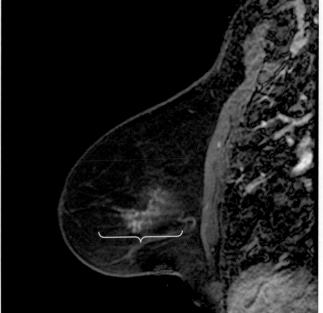

Plate 7.5F

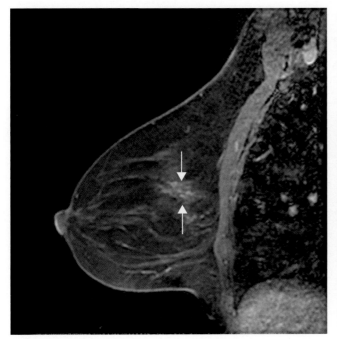

Plate 7.5G

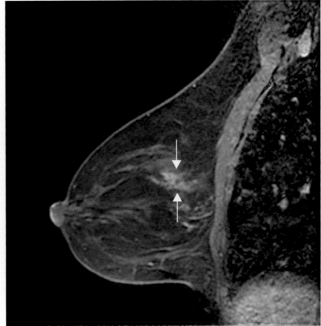

Plate 7.5H

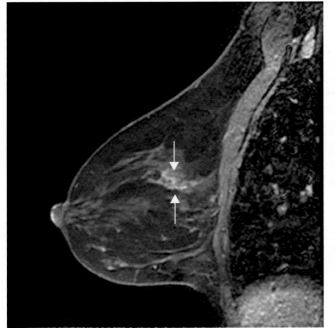

Plate 7.5I

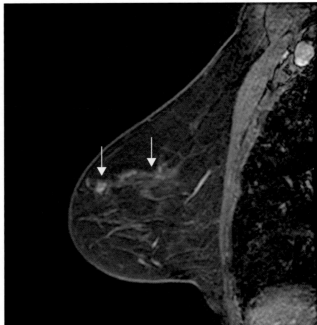

Plate 7.5J

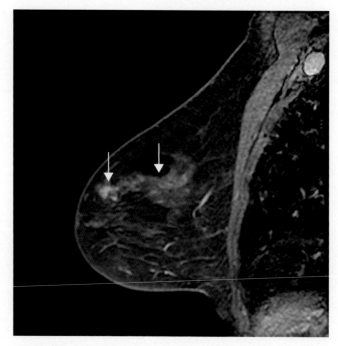

Plate 7.5K

FINDINGS

- Plates 7.5A–D—Digital mammography demonstrating mixed fibroglandular and fatty tissue with mildly asymmetric tissue in the right upper outer breast and scattered calcifications, unchanged from previous exams.

- Plates 7.5E–F—Postcontrast series, demonstrating a large area of clumped enhancement (3:00 axis) and grouped enhancing foci. There is also linear enhancement extending anteriorly towards the nipple, highly suggestive of DCIS.

- Plates 7.5G–I—Demonstrate linear and grouped progressively enhancing foci in the 12:00 axis, which also proved on biopsy to represent DCIS.

- Plates 7.5J–K—Demonstrate a small area of nodular/clumped enhancement in the right upper outer quadrant, which was also evaluated with core biopsy. It was found to represent only fibrocystic changes on MRI core biopsy.

DISCUSSION

Not every suspicious area will be a carcinoma; in cases with multiple areas of concern in an extent of disease workup, choose the most suspicious area to biopsy first. If this area proves benign, the remaining less suspicious appearing areas are also likely to be benign and can be safely followed. However, in cases of highly suspicious finding (e.g. spiculated mass, irregular linear enhancement), a benign biopsy result should be considered discordant, and excisional biopsy should proceed.

• **Plate 6**

HISTORY

49-year-old woman who presented with an area of tenderness in the left upper breast with no palpable mass on physical exam. Bilateral mammogram and ultrasound demonstrated smooth nodules, consistent with cysts, but no suspicious masses. MRI was done for clinical problem solving.

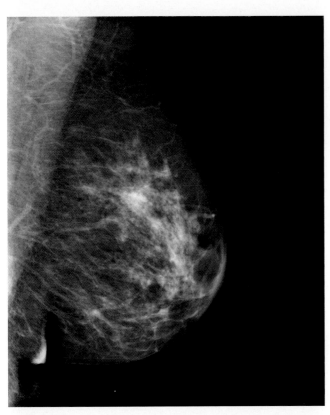

Plate 7.6A

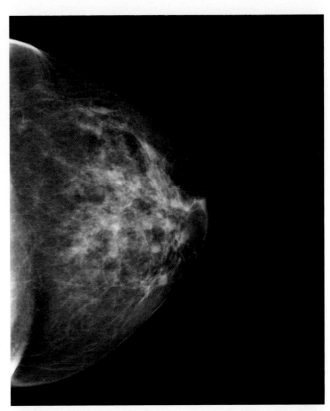

Plate 7.6B

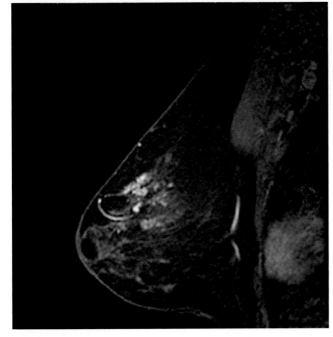

Plate 7.6C

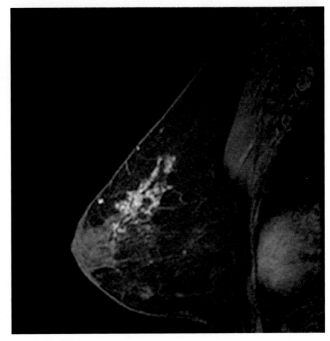

Plate 7.6D

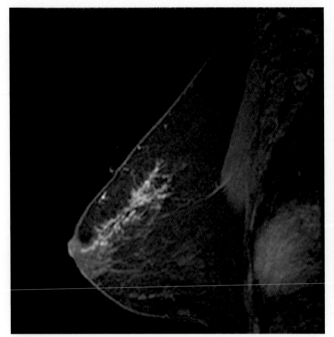

Plate 7.6E

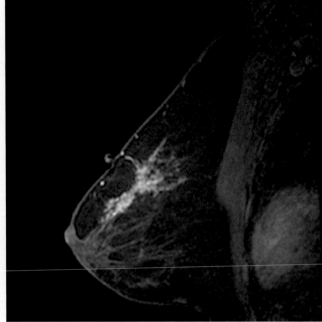

Plate 7.6F

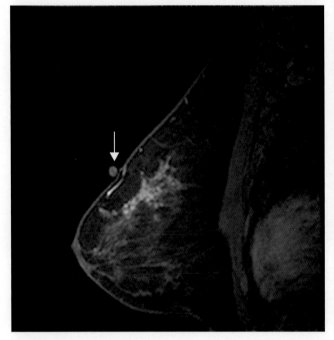

Plate 7.6G

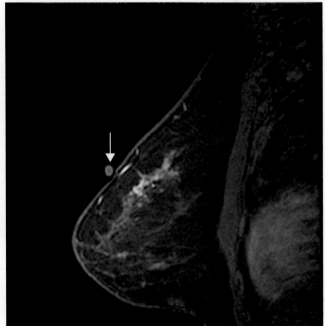

Plate 7.6H

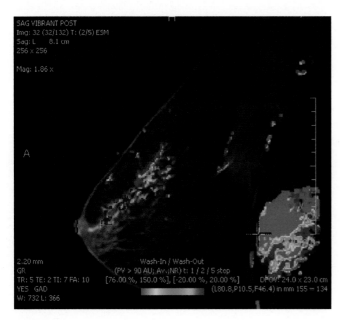

Plate 7.6I

FINDINGS

- Plates 7.6A–B—Bilateral digital screening digital mammography had demonstrated benign-appearing nodules found to correspond to cysts on ultrasound and heterogeneously dense parenchyma.

- Plates 7.6C–H—Numerous sections extending from the 10:00 to 2:00 axis with extensive linear and clumped enhancement in a segmental distribution, highly suggestive of DCIS, with linear enhancement extending into the nipple. Note the vitamin E capsule, which corresponds to patient's area of symptomatology (pain). The enhancement kinetics are very heterogeneous, but predominantly progressive and plateau.

DISCUSSION

MRI core biopsies were done at the anterior and posterior aspects of the lesion, which both demonstrated DCIS. Patient desired breast conservation despite recommendation for mastectomy, and therefore the area was bracketed for attempted lumpectomy. Final pathology yielded 8.0 cm of intermediate DCIS with foci of microinvasion. Margins were positive, and she ultimately underwent a mastectomy. With this large area of involvement on MRI, and disease documented with positive core biopsy at anterior and posterior extents, obtaining clear margins at lumpectomy is unlikely. If this was attempted, the cosmetic result would likely be unacceptable.

• CASE 1

HISTORY

A 60-year-old woman presented with routine screening mammogram with a large stellate left upper outer quadrant asymmetric density and no corresponding physical findings.

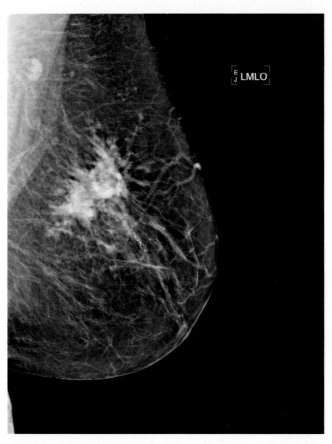

Figure 8.1A

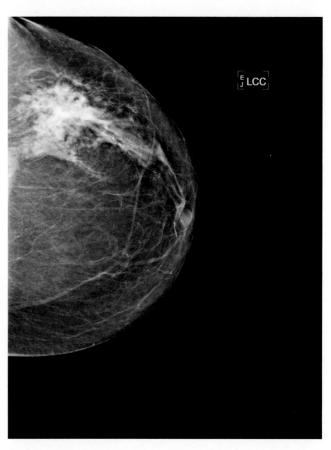

Figure 8.1B

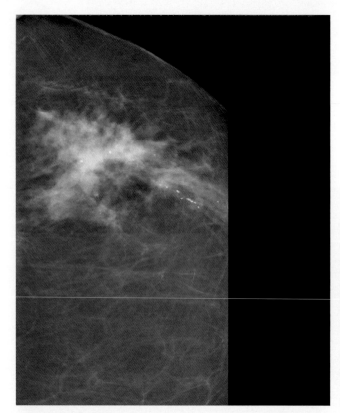

Figure 8.1C

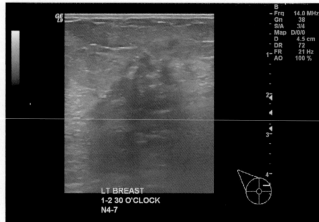

Figure 8.1D

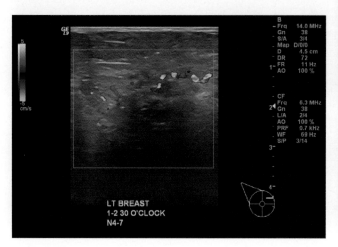

Figure 8.1E

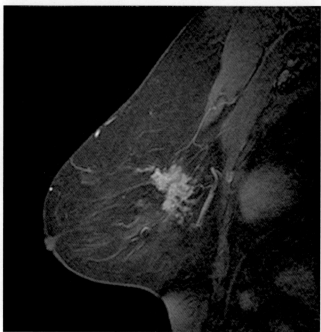

Figure 8.1F

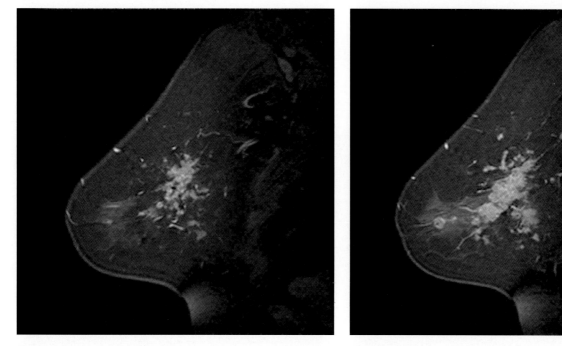

Figure 8.1G

Figure 8.1H

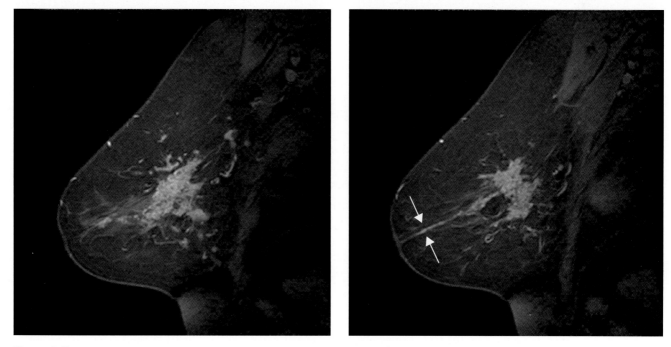

Figure 8.1I

Figure 8.1J

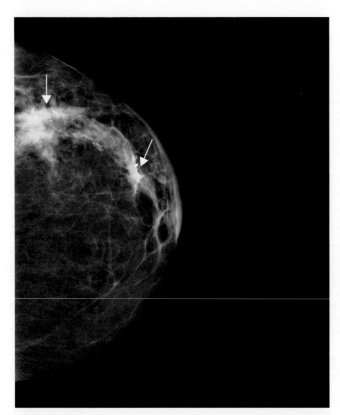

Figure 8.1K

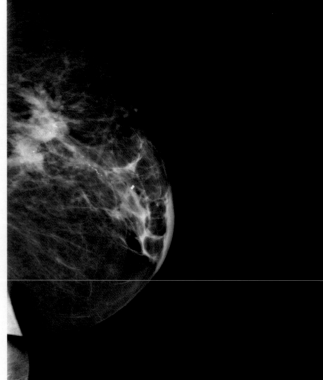

Figure 8.1L

FINDINGS

- Figures 8.1A–C—Digital mammogram demonstrating a spiculated irregular left upper outer quadrant mass with pleomorphic calcifications as well as several ductal type of calcifications extending anteriorly towards the nipple.

- Figures 8.1D–E—Ultrasound (US) demonstrating a large poorly defined area of shadowing and hypoechogenicity with increased vascularity.

- Figure 8.1F—Magnetic resonance imaging (MRI) demonstrates the spiculated enhancing mass in the posterior left upper outer quadrant.

- Figures 8.1G–J—Additional areas of nodular, clumped, and linear enhancement as well as small enhancing masses are present throughout the left upper outer quadrant. Linear enhancement extending towards the nipple (Fig. 8.1J) is characteristic of ductal carcinoma in situ (DCIS).

- Figures 8.1K–L—Digital mammogram after two biopsies, the clip from the US-guided biopsy is in the posterior mass, and the second clip from the MRI-guided biopsy is in the anterior area of the breast (periareolar) at site of linear enhancement.

WORKUP

- An US-guided core biopsy was performed and demonstrated invasive carcinoma. MRI was performed for extent of disease evaluation. On MRI, there is an irregular spiculated enhancing left upper quadrant mass, additional clumped linear and nodular enhancement, as well as other satellite enhancing nodules spanning an area of >10 cm. A second biopsy was performed of the anterior extent of linear enhancement to document the extent of disease. This demonstrated additional disease with a focus of DCIS and invasive carcinoma, 8 cm from the original clip.

DISCUSSION

Even when mammographic findings are obvious, we perform extent of disease evaluation because unsuspected additional disease can still be revealed on MRI. The size of tumor involvement on MRI was approximately twice the size of the suspected disease based on mammographic or sonographic findings. For the clinicians, this allows for a more thorough evaluation for consideration of neoadjuvant therapy, as well as information necessary to decide between mastectomy and breast conservation. After initial diagnosis, if the tumor size appears significantly larger/more extensive, a second biopsy should be performed to confirm the imaging findings. Choose an area furthest away from the first clip. As a general rule, tumor involvement greater than 5 cm prompts mastectomy as the treatment of choice instead of lumpectomy. This rule of thumb varies with breast size, because a large breast may be able to accommodate a larger resection with a reasonable cosmetic result. This should be decided in discussion with the surgeon.

Even if the patient is electing mastectomy, it is wise to document the extent of tumor as the patient may have second thoughts after mastectomy. The second biopsy with clip placement also helps the pathologist to locate this site, which may otherwise be difficult to find in a large mastectomy specimen. The pathologist is unlikely to find a small focus of DCIS away from the known carcinoma, unless a clip is present and the pathologist is made aware of the documented presence of multifocal/multicentric synchronous disease.

• CASE 2

HISTORY

A 71-year-old woman with a family history of two daughters with premenopausal breast cancer, who had not had a mammogram in 2 years, presents for mammographic evaluation. Her screening mammogram demonstrated a new left breast mass.

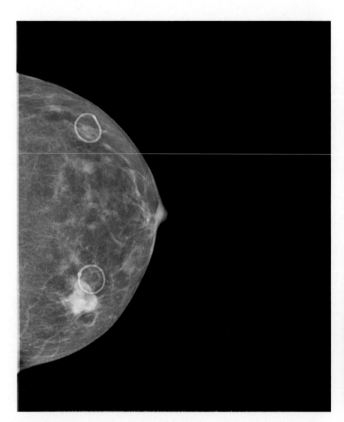

Figure 8.2A

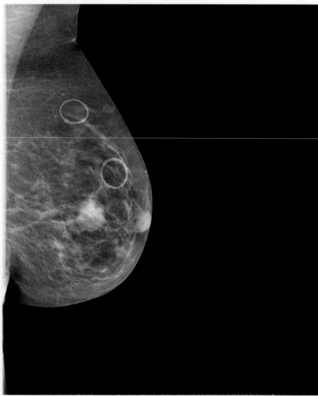

Figure 8.2B

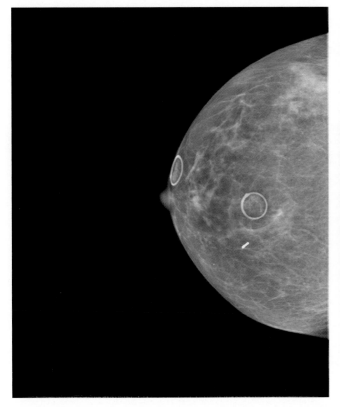

Figure 8.2C

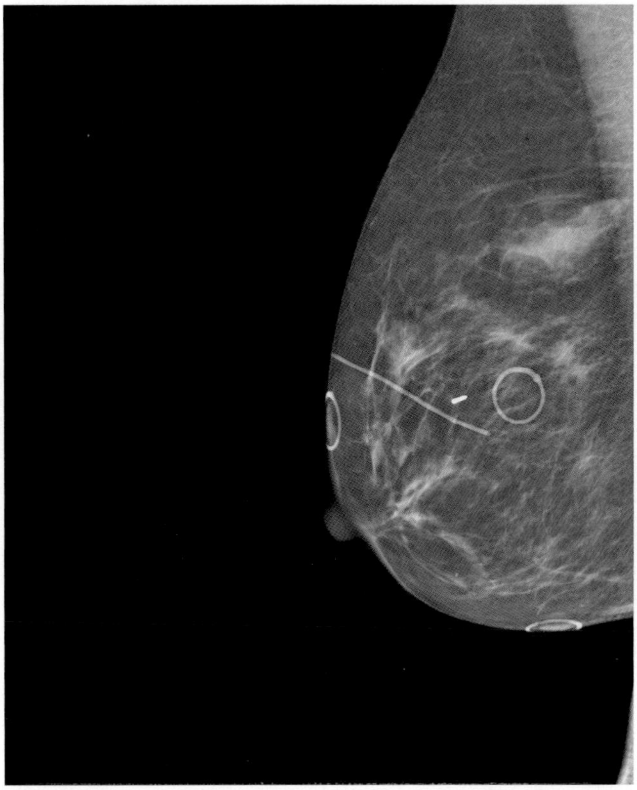

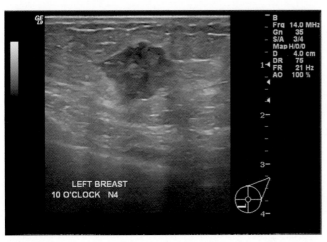

Figure 8.2E

Figure 8.2D

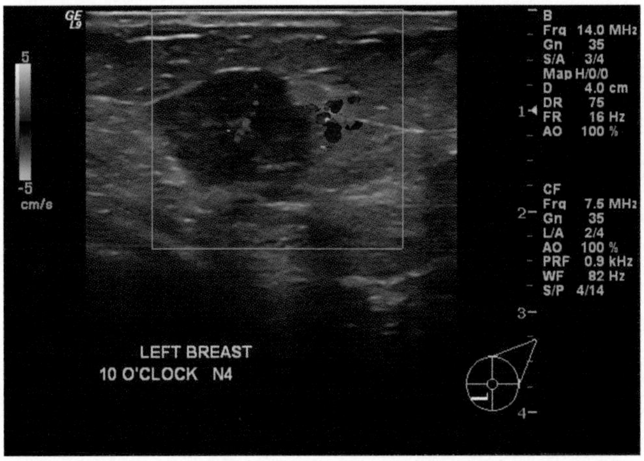

Figure 8.2F

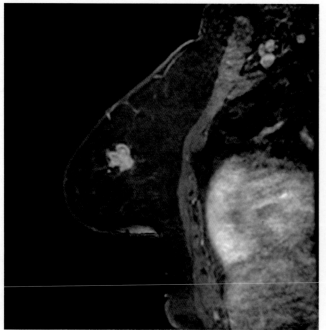

Figure 8.2G

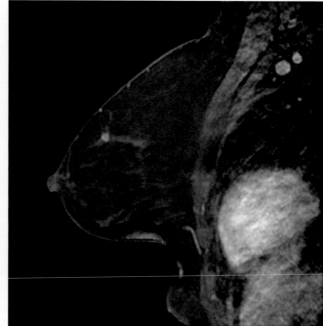

Figure 8.2H

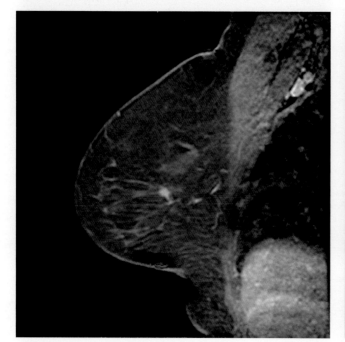

Figure 8.2I

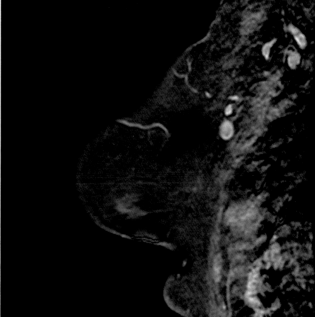

Figure 8.2J

FINDINGS

- Figures 8.2A–B—Demonstrates the initial screening mammogram with a suspicious 1.9-cm mass left mass with indistinct and irregular margins.

- Figures 8.2C–D—Digital mammographic images demonstrating right breast with a mole marker in place, a clip from prior benign biopsy, and skin marker over prior benign surgical biopsy scar. The breast parenchyma is relatively fatty, and no suspicious findings are seen.

- Figures 8.2E–F—Demonstrate a heterogeneous left inner upper quadrant hypoechoic mass with internal vascularity. Some of the margin is well circumscribed, whereas the other areas are irregular/indistinct and lobulated. This corresponds to the mammographic findings. Increased flow is noted.

- Figure 8.2G—A sagittal postcontrast image, demonstrating a lobulated ring enhancing mass that is characteristic of carcinoma, corresponding to the mammographic/sonographic findings.

- Figure 8.2H—Demonstrates a second smaller enhancing mass in the 12:00 axis of the left breast.

- Figure 8.2I—A third, small enhancing mass with radiating spicules with adjacent linear enhancement is seen in the right outer breast.

- Figure 8.2J—Demonstrates an abnormal left axillary lymph node, which is rounded and has lost its normal fatty hilum.

WORKUP

- US-guided core biopsy was performed and demonstrated invasive ductal carcinoma. MRI is performed for extent of disease evaluation. In addition to the known carcinoma in the left inner breast, a second small enhancing mass was seen in the left 12:00 axis, and third mass is seen at the right breast 9:00 axis. Also noted were prominent lymph nodes in the left axilla. MRI core biopsies were performed. The right breast demonstrated invasive ductal carcinoma. The left 12:00 axis nodule also demonstrated invasive carcinoma. Fine-needle aspiration biopsy of left axillary node was positive for metastatic disease.

DISCUSSION

In this case, a woman with relatively fatty breasts was going to undergoing lumpectomy for a new left mass detected on screening. On MRI, multicentric disease is seen in the left breast as well as synchronous contralateral carcinoma in the right breast. Both of these additional findings would have gone undetected without MRI and would likely have resulted in treatment failure.

Even though she and her daughters have breast cancer, they are BRCA-negative. There are families with genetic risk other than the BRCA 1 and 2 genes.

The abnormal lymph noted followed by fine-needle aspiration biopsy of this node saved the additional procedure of sentinel node biopsy, and assisted with surgical planning.

• CASE 3

HISTORY

A 56-year-old woman who presented with an abnormal screening mammogram that demonstrated a small new nodule (4 mm).

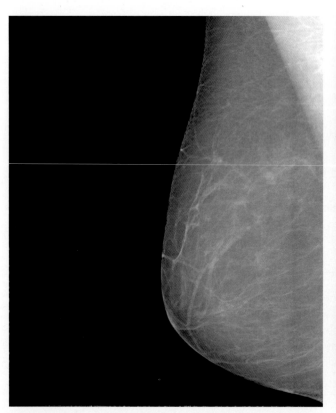

Figure 8.3A

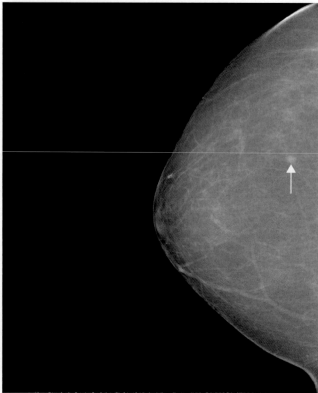

Figure 8.3B

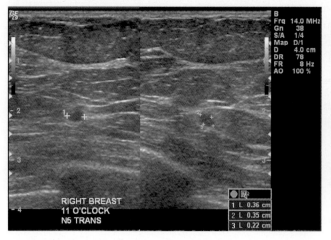

Figure 8.3C

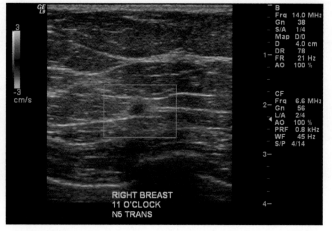

Figure 8.3D

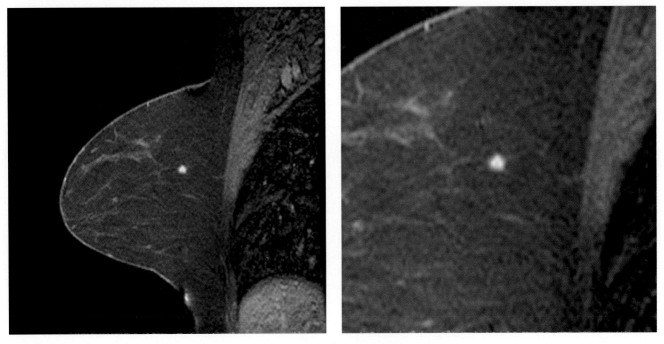

Figure 8.3E

Figure 8.3F

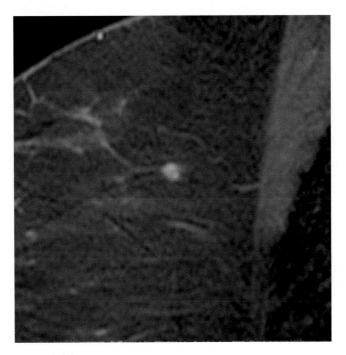

Figure 8.3G

FINDINGS

- Figures 8.3A–B—Screening mammogram with a new 4-mm density in the right upper posterior breast. It appears smooth on the mediolateral oblique view but does appear slightly spiculated in the craniocaudal view.
- Figures 8.3C–D—US demonstrating a tiny hypoechoic nodule 1, which could be mistaken for a small complicated cyst. There is however a suggestion of a thickened rind.
- Figure 8.3E—MRI with an intensely enhancing 4-mm nodule in the corresponding location.
- Figure 8.3F—A magnified image of MRI demonstrates the margins are somewhat angular. This nodule is so small that characteristic features of carcinoma are hard to appreciate. It did, however, demonstrate washout enhancement kinetics.
- Figure 8.3G—A more delayed image with decreased enhancement and central clearing indicating subtle washout and ring enhancement.

WORKUP

- MRI scan was recommended for mammographic problem solving, because the nodule was too small to target for stereotactic biopsy and initial US was negative. MRI scan demonstrated an intensely enhancing focus with areas of washout kinetics and slightly irregular margins. Repeat targeted US was preformed and demonstrated a 3.5-mm hypoechoic nodule; biopsy was performed and demonstrated invasive ductal carcinoma. The remainder of the MRI demonstrated no other disease. Lumpectomy with sentinel node biopsy was performed. Final pathology demonstrated minute foci of residual carcinoma.

DISCUSSION

Ideally, because this nodule represented a new mammographic finding that could not be demonstrated to represent a simple cyst, it should have been biopsied with stereotactic guidance. (The BIRADS designation should have been "4") If stereotactic biopsy was not available, excisional biopsy should have been performed.

If you have a finding that is indeterminate or frankly suspicious on mammogram or ultrasound, MRI should not be used to shortcut the appropriate workup. A new nodule in a postmenopausal woman on a mammogram that does not prove to be a cyst warrants a biopsy even if there was no enhancement on MRI. There are occasional times when an MRI will demonstrate a benign structure, and can prevent an unnecessary biopsy, such as MRI demonstrating a corresponding intramammary lymph node, fat necrosis, or complex cyst with no enhancement. If the MRI fails to find a definitive diagnosis, then proceed to work up the abnormality, by sampling (needle biopsy or excisional biopsy if necessary). In this case, the MRI, although not truly necessary to evaluate the mammographic nodule, would have been done anyway as part of her extent of disease evaluation.

Ideally, a breast surgeon will take the patient to the operating room *after* the diagnosis has been established with needle biopsy. The surgical planning for a lumpectomy is different than for an excisional biopsy, and even BIRADS 5 lesions should have needle biopsy–proven pathology before going to the operating room. Even if a radiologic abnormality is scheduled to be localized/excised, attempt core biopsy first.

• CASE 4

HISTORY

A 44-year-old woman with complaint of a palpable abnormality in the left breast at an outside clinic for 1 year. Outside digital mammography and sonography had been negative, and surgical or needle biopsy was not performed.

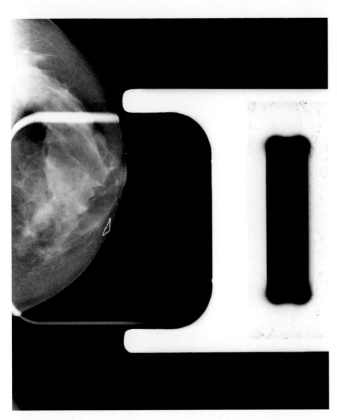

Figure 8.4A

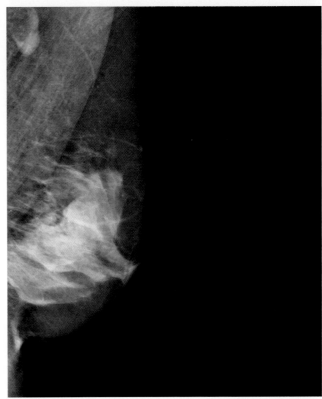

Figure 8.4B

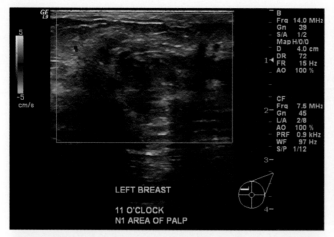

Figure 8.4C

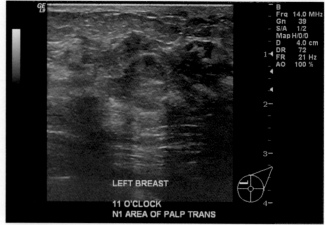

Figure 8.4D

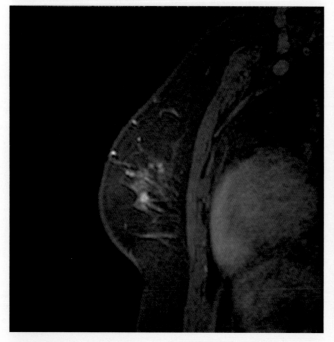

Figure 8.4E

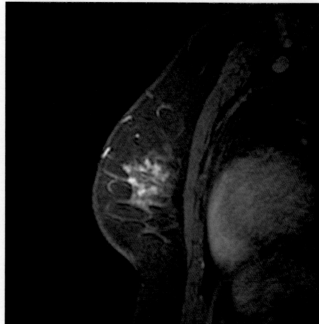

Figure 8.4F

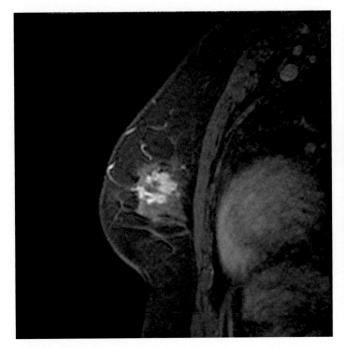

Figure 8.4G

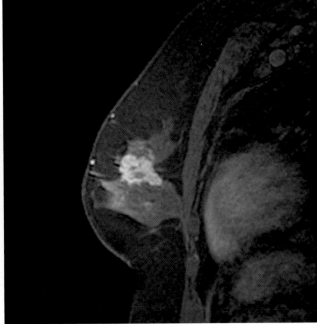

Figure 8.4H

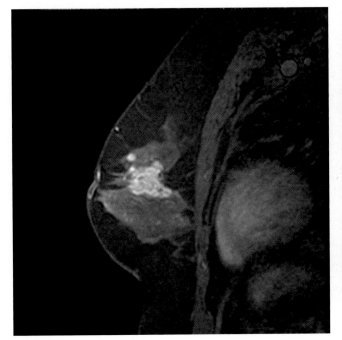

Figure 8.4I

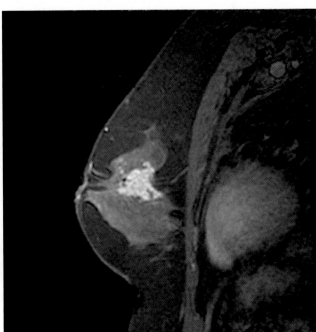

Figure 8.4J

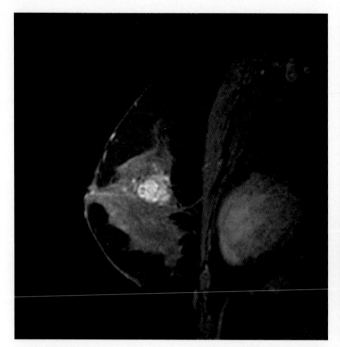

Figure 8.4K

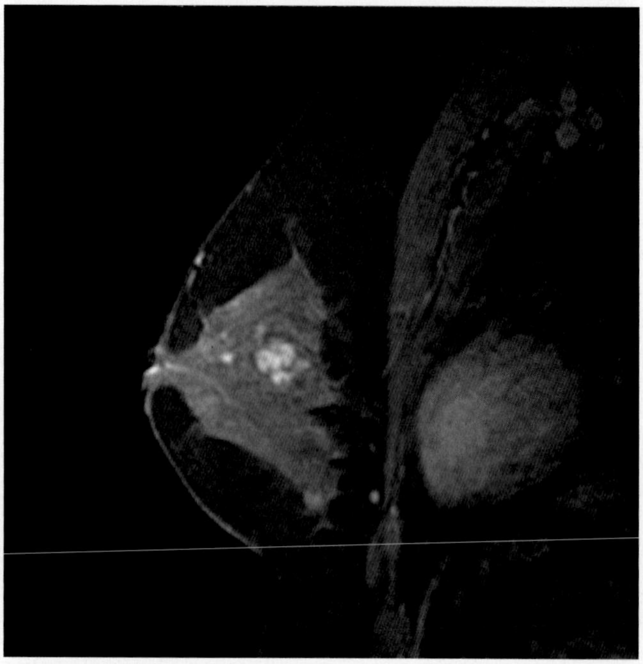

Figure 8.4L

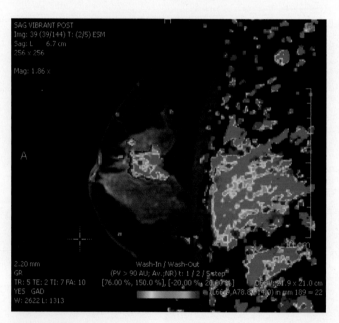

Figure 8.4M

FINDINGS

- Figures 8.4 A–B—Demonstrates a dense breast with some mildly asymmetric soft-tissue density corresponding to the palpable abnormality, as indicated by the triangular marker over the area of concern.
- Figures 8.4C–D—US demonstrating a hypoechoic lobulated mass with enhanced through transmission.
- Figures 8.4E–M—Serial sagittal postcontrast images demonstrating a large enhancing irregular mass with multiple satellite nodules, and linear enhancement extending toward the nipple.
- Note the heterogeneous enhancement kinetics including areas of washout with satellite nodule superiorly with same kinetics pattern.

WORKUP

- She presented to our facility for evaluation/second opinion. US-guided core biopsy was performed and demonstrated presence of invasive ductal carcinoma. MRI was performed for extent of disease evaluation. On MRI, a 3-cm left breast mass was noted with surrounding enhancing nodules and evidence of left axillary adenopathy. She subsequently underwent a mastectomy. Final pathology demonstrated 3.3-cm invasive ductal, associated extensive DCIS and 6/18 positive axillary nodes.

DISCUSSION

This is an unfortunate case of a reportedly negative outside digital mammography and sonography resulting in an incomplete workup of a palpable mass. As radiologists know, a negative digital mammography or sonography should not prevent biopsy of a clinically suspicious palpable mass. This is a major cause of "delay in diagnosis."

This patient had no elevated risk factors other than extremely dense parenchyma. It is obvious from the MRI findings that this mass would have been clearly visible on MRI at even a quarter of the size at which it presented. We perform MRI scans for unexplained clinical findings with negative digital mammography and sonography. Although this lesion should have been excised with or without suspicious MRI findings, a preoperative MRI demonstrating the abnormal area allows for targeting and preoperative core biopsy. Subsequent definitive surgery/oncologic treatment can then be performed (e.g., neoadjuvant chemotherapy). When the extent of the disease is large, biopsy of more than one area is recommended.

• CASE 5

HISTORY

A 37-year-old woman presented with a palpable right breast mass. She has no notable risk factors.

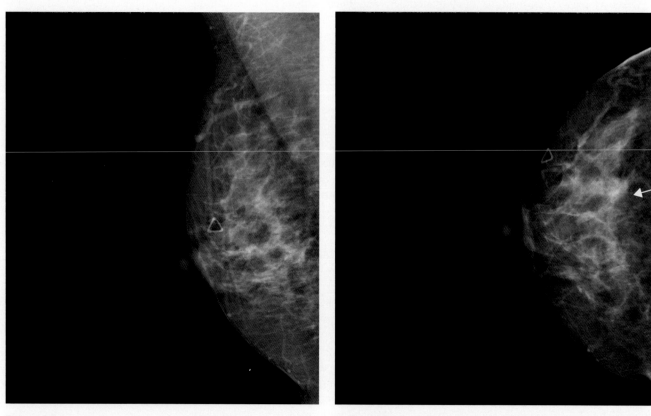

Figure 8.5A   Figure 8.5B

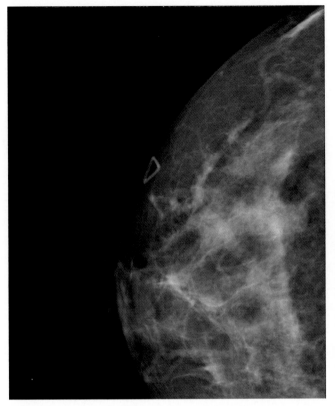

Figure 8.5C

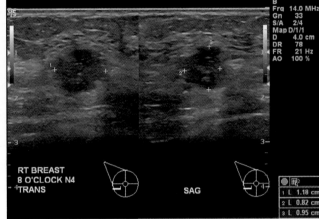

Figure 8.5D

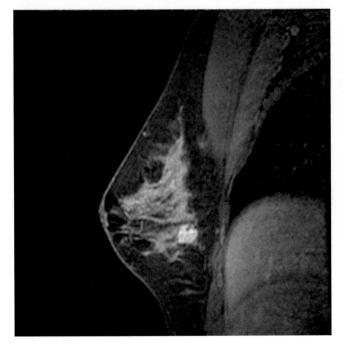

Figure 8.5E

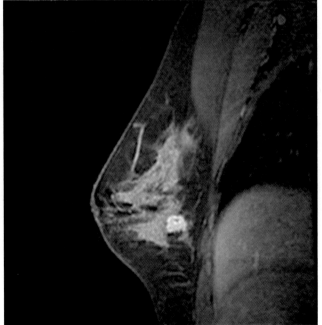

Figure 8.5F

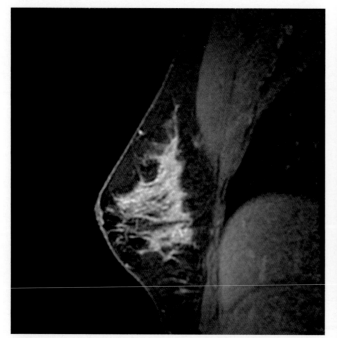

Figure 8.5G

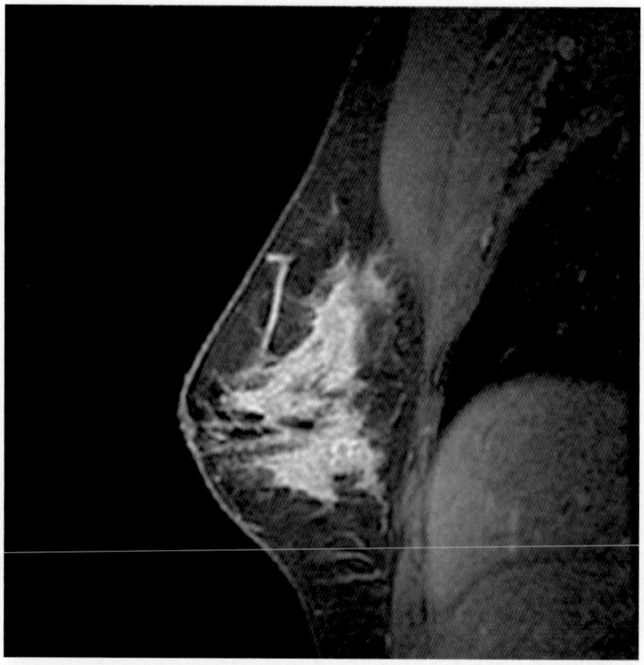

Figure 8.5H

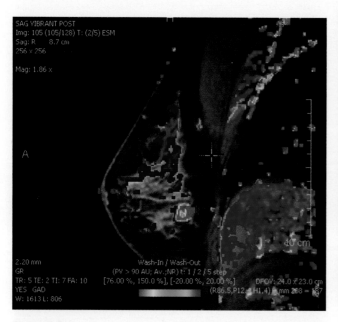

Figure 8.5I

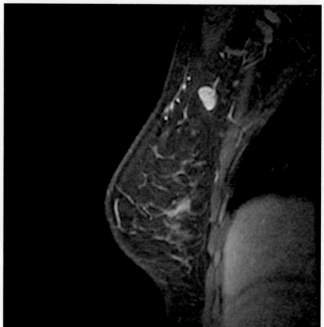

Figure 8.5J

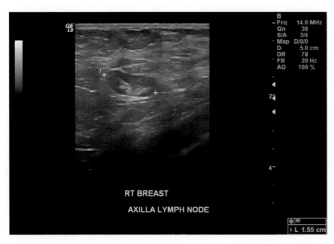

Figure 8.5K

FINDINGS

- Figures 8.5A–C—A digital right breast image demonstrating heterogeneously dense parenchyma with a 1.5-cm asymmetric nodular density deep to the palpable marker (arrow), containing some ductal, "branching" suspicious calcifications.

- Figure 8.5D—Sonographic images demonstrating a poorly defined irregular hypoechoic mass measuring 1.3 cm, containing calcifications. The margin features are suspicious for malignancy but enhanced through transmission is noted.

- Figures 8.5E–F—Sagittal images from the first postcontrast series demonstrating a 1.3 cm slightly irregular ring enhancing mass containing the metallic clip from core biopsy.

- Figures 8.5G–H—The corresponding fourth postcontrast series. In this case, because of the markedly large component of washout enhancement kinetics and the severe background enhancement, the mass is *less* conspicuous on the delayed images.

- Figure 8.5I—Enhancement kinetics are heterogeneously, but predominantly washout. Also note the severe progressive background enhancement, seen best in the upper breast on this particular image.

- Figure 8.5J—MRI postcontrast image depicting an abnormal appearing lymph node. Note the absence of normal fatty hilum and its prominent size.

- Figure 8.5K—Demonstrate targeted US of an axillary lymph node with thickened cortex. This was found to contain metastatic ductal cancer on fine-needle aspiration biopsy.

WORKUP

- An US core needle biopsy was recommended and was positive for invasive ductal carcinoma. She had an MRI, which demonstrated a well-defined enhancing mass with marked washout kinetics. An enlarged axillary lymph node was also noted. Otherwise no evidence of synchronous disease was seen.

DISCUSSION

Because of the classic washout enhancement kinetics combined with the marked background enhancement on MRI, this lesion is less visible on delayed images. It is important to image quickly after power injection of contrast. As the background enhancement increases the lesion is more obscured. The only feature that becomes more prominent on the later images is the ring enhancement. In our experience, the majority of all malignant lesions, including invasive and in situ ductal and lobular, carcinomas have more areas that are progressively enhancing than areas that are "washing out." In other words, most malignancies have not "read the textbook." However, the majority of invasive ductal carcinomas that are larger than 1 cm do contain some areas with washout enhancement kinetics.

Although this woman had no risk factors, she presented with breast cancer at an early age. It is important to remember that the majority of breast cancer patients do *not* have a positive family history, and the patient and clinician may need to be reminded of this as well.

In this case, aside from the enlarged lymph node and the known carcinoma, the MRI was negative. When we see a suspicious lymph node on MRI, we bring patients back for targeted US and possible fine needle aspiration. If this node is found to be positive, we can avoid the additional surgical procedure of sentinel node biopsy and the surgeon will usually go directly to axillary dissection at the time of lumpectomy or mastectomy. If it is negative, then sentinel node biopsy is still performed.

No solitary feature of a lesion should persuade you to ignore other suspicious features. In this case on the US, one of the features (enhanced through transmission) suggests benign disease; however, it is not uncommon for carcinomas to present this way. This reflects a homogeneous tumor cell population.

• CASE 6

HISTORY

A 44-year-old woman with strongly positive family history of breast cancer. She had a negative bilateral screening digital mammography and was referred for breast MRI for high-risk screening.

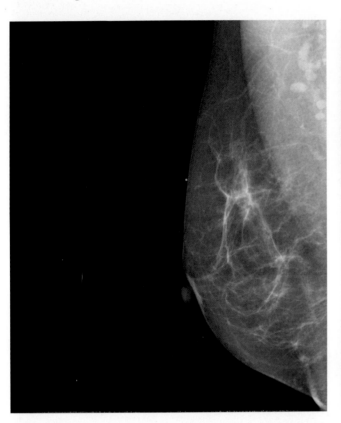

Figure 8.6A

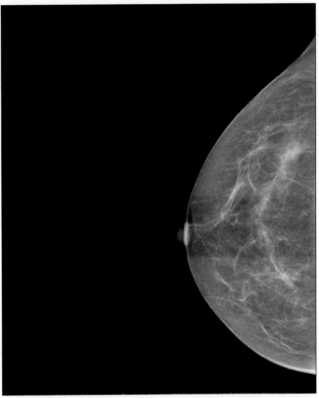

Figure 8.6B

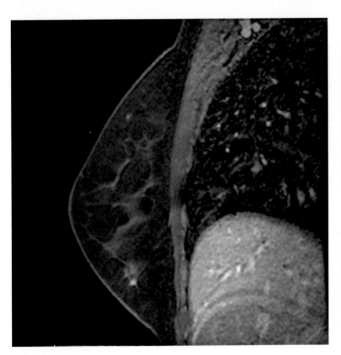

Figure 8.6C

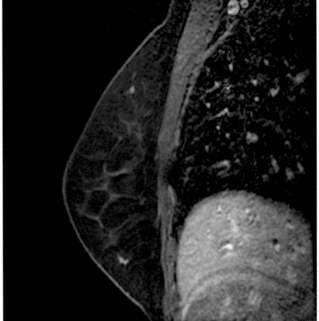

Figure 8.6D

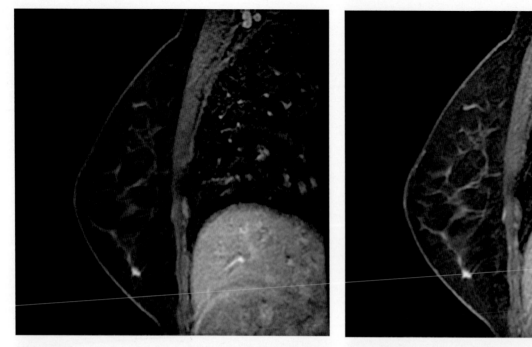

Figure 8.6E

Figure 8.6F

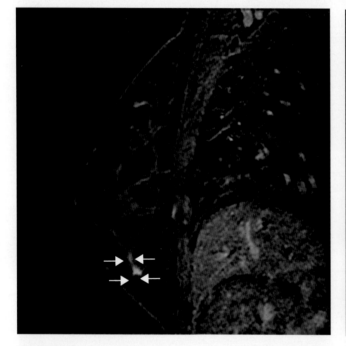

Figure 8.6G

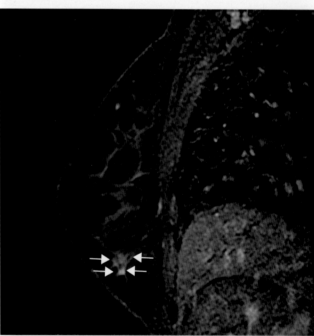

Figure 8.6H

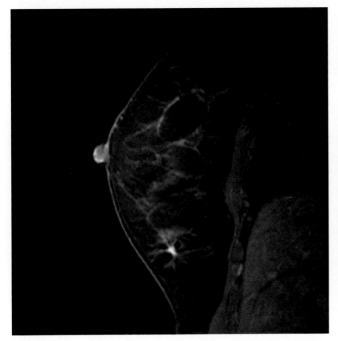

Figure 8.6I

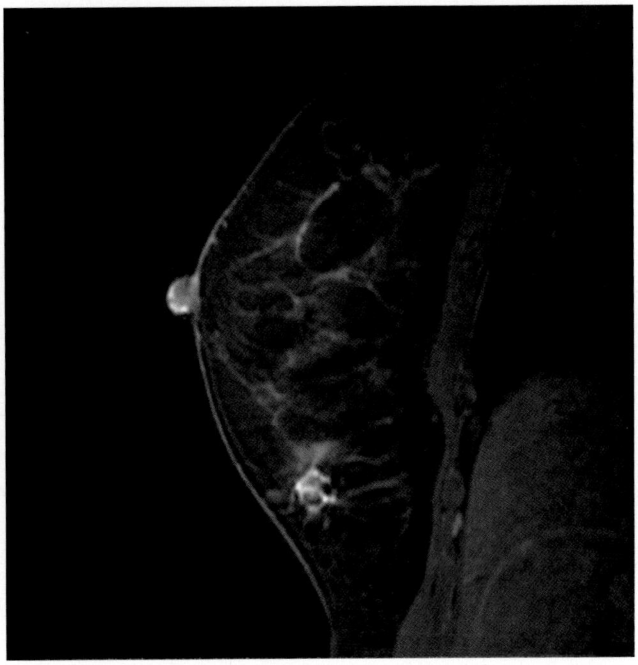

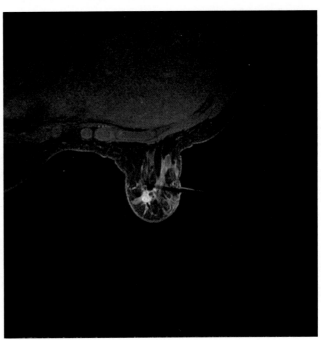

Figure 8.6J

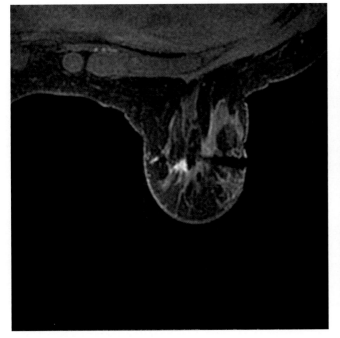

Figure 8.6K

Figure 8.6L

FINDINGS

- Figures 8.6A–B—Demonstrate bilateral screening digital mammography with predominantly fatty breasts with no masses, calcifications, or interval changes from prior exams.
- Figures 8.6C–E—Demonstrate sagittal postcontrast images a 6 × 4 mm irregular nodule with an adjacent enhancing focus in the 5:00 to 6:00 axis of the right breast.
- Figure 8.6F—Fourth postcontrast series, which demonstrates increased background enhancement with the suspicious nodule appearing slightly larger and more prominent (i.e., progressive enhancement kinetics).
- Figures 8.6G–H—Subtracted series shows the conspicuous enhancing nodule with some adjacent (superior) enhancement, which is suspicious for surrounding DCIS (arrow).
- Figure 8.6I,K—Demonstrate images from MRI core biopsy, axial and sagittal, with satisfactory needle placement.
- Figure 8.6J,L—Postbiopsy sagittal and axial view.

WORKUP

- An enhancing lesion was seen on the MRI in the right lower breast. MRI core biopsy was performed and demonstrated invasive ductal carcinoma.

DISCUSSION

The core biopsy results demonstrated both invasive ductal carcinoma and DCIS. Even though this woman has fatty breasts on digital mammography, the lesion is not appreciable even in retrospect. In a lesion as small as this, we would not recommend attempting targeted US, because it may delay the definitive biopsy. US is also less likely to be helpful when the breast parenchyma is fatty.

When performing MRI-guided core biopsy always confirm that the lesion has been adequately sampled. We do this by comparing the sagittal image with the lesion and the needle pre biopsy and the corresponding postbiopsy image to ensure that at least part of the lesion is no longer visible. If there is any question, we perform an axial series, demonstrating that postbiopsy cavity is now present in the exact position where the lesion was previously seen.

Clip placement is essential in MRI core biopsy, so that future procedures such as localization can be performed with mammographic instead of MRI guidance.

• Plate 1

HISTORY

A 67-year-old woman presented with a new nodule on screening digital mammography. This was found on US to correspond to an irregular hypoechoic lesion with increased vascularity. An US-guided core biopsy was performed and demonstrated the presence of poorly differentiated neuroendocrine small cell type carcinoma. She underwent MRI, which demonstrates no additional suspicious findings. Preoperative workup to exclude a lung primary was also negative. She subsequently underwent lumpectomy. Final pathology demonstrated a 1.1-cm undifferentiated carcinoma with neuroendocrine features with DCIS. This case is included to demonstrate that invasive ductal carcinomas can have unusual pathologic features, even when the imaging findings relatively classic for carcinoma. In such cases, the workup and treatment of breast carcinoma should not be impeded by unusual pathologic features.

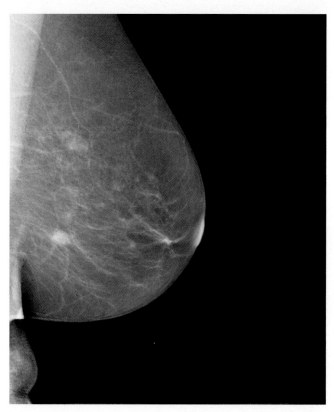

Plate 8.1A

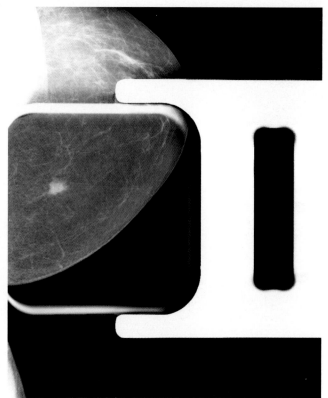

Plate 8.1B

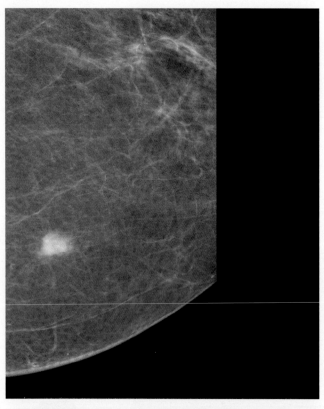

Plate 8.1C

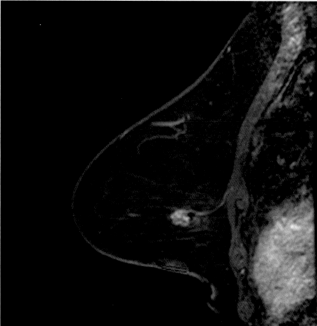

LT BREAST

9 O'CLOCK N7 SAG

Plate 8.1D

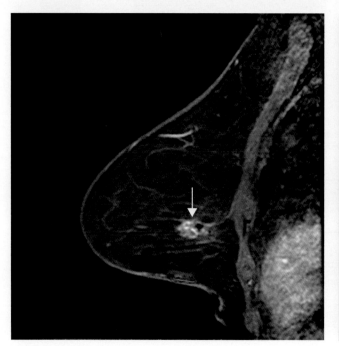

Plate 8.1E

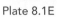

Plate 8.1F

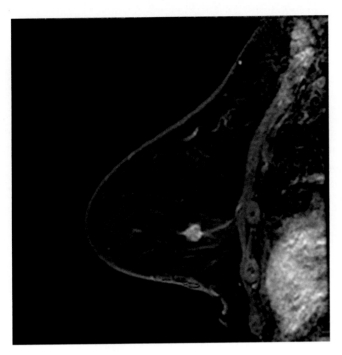

Plate 8.1G

FINDINGS

- Plates 8.1A–C—Demonstrate digital mammographic images a 1.1-cm mass with some irregular and indistinct margins and microcalcifications.

- Plate 8.1D—Hypoechoic mass on ultrasound with internal vascularity and very irregular nodular, lobulated margins.

- Plates 8.1E–G—Demonstrate postcontrast sagittal series, depicting a lobulated 1.2-cm mass with ring enhancement, and some slightly spiculated and nodular margins. Also seen is the adjacent metallic clip that was placed at time of the US-guided core biopsy.

- Note the "feeding vessel" posteriorly. This is commonly seen with invasive carcinomas and must be distinguished from linear extension/DCIS. A vessel is traceable anteriorly and posteriorly on contiguous slices. Vessels can be seen to penetrate the pectoral muscle, and then usually become oriented superiorly or inferiorly.

• Plate 2

HISTORY

A 61-year-old woman presented with an area of increased density in the right upper outer quadrant on screening digital mammography. Additional views and US confirm the presence of a poorly defined hypoechoic mass measuring approximately 2 cm. Incidentally noted is a nearby 1-cm benign-appearing nodule, which was subsequently aspirated and found to represent a debris-filled cyst. She had an US-guided core biopsy of the solid mass, which demonstrated invasive ductal carcinoma. An MRI scan was performed for extent of disease and demonstrated a 2.5-cm enhancing irregular and spiculated mass consistent with the known carcinoma. Despite the large tumor size in this patient, the axillary lymph nodes appeared normal. She underwent lumpectomy and axillary evaluation and was found to have no axillary disease at final pathology.

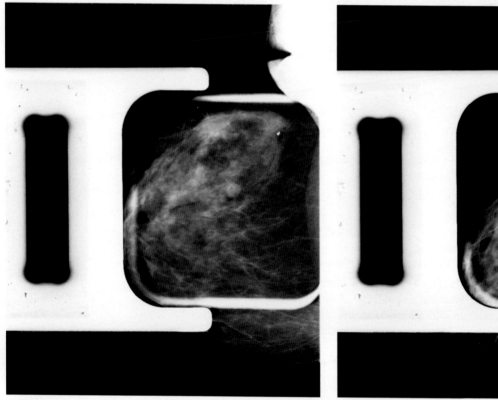

Plate 8.2A

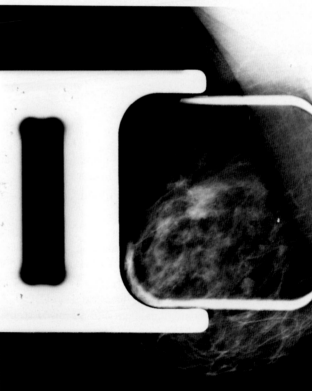

Plate 8.2B

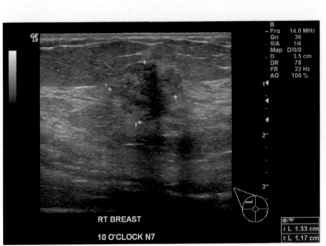

Plate 8.2C

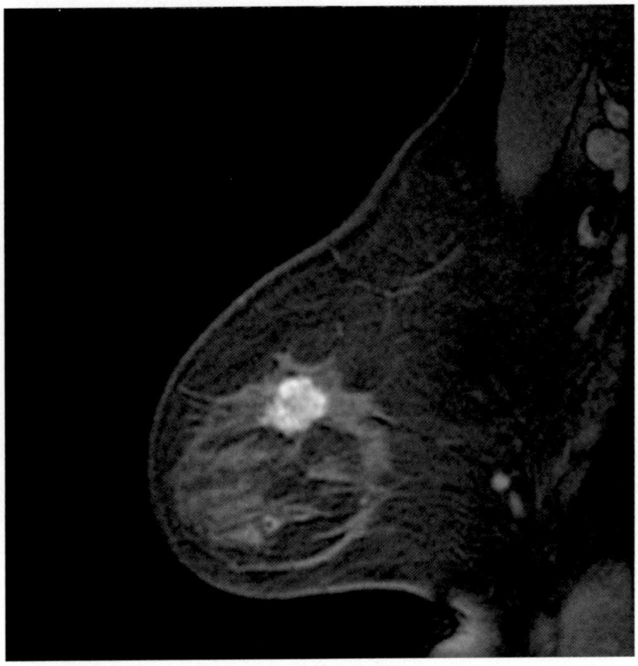

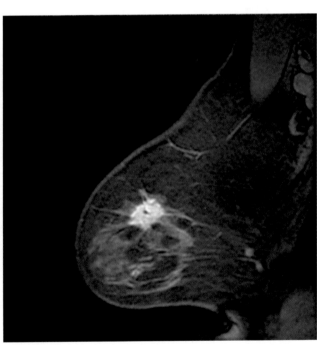

Plate 8.2D

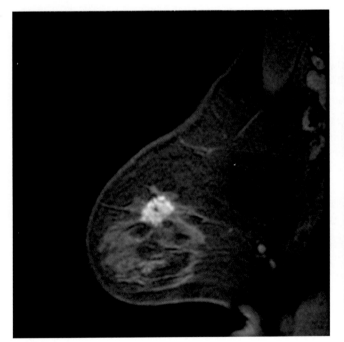

Plate 8.2E

Plate 8.2F

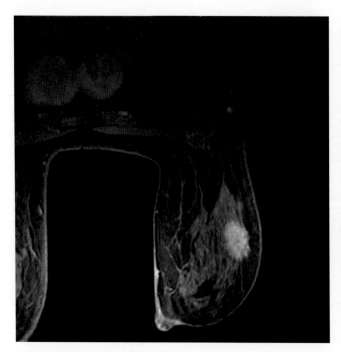

Plate 8.2G

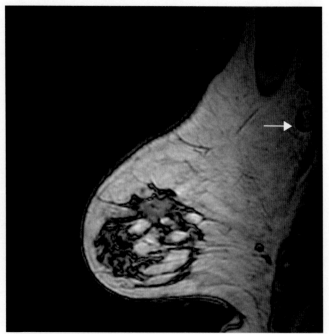

Plate 8.2H

FINDINGS

- Plates 8.2A–B—Demonstrate spot views from a digital mammogram with dense parenchyma and a poorly defined nodule in the upper most, outer most region. A 1-cm smooth well defined nodule is seen more centrally.

- Plate 8.2C—Demonstrates the poorly defined irregular hypoechoic shadowing structure corresponding to the larger mass.

- Plates 8.2D–F—Sagittal images demonstrating a 2.5-cm irregular enhancing mass with spiculations and with heterogeneous internal enhancement. The spiculations become more evident on the fourth series (D). The mass contains the clip placed at the time of US guided core biopsy.

- Plate 8.2G—Delayed axial image. The obvious enhancing mass is seen and the spiculations have become very evident.

- Plate 8.2H—Demonstrates the normal-appearing axillary lymph node with thin cortex and fatty hilum.

• Plate 3

HISTORY

A 52-year-old woman presented with a palpable left breast mass found to correspond to a spiculated mass in the left outer lower breast quadrant on digital mammography. US demonstrated the presence of a corresponding irregular mass with increased vascularity. A US core biopsy was performed and demonstrated an invasive ductal carcinoma. MRI was performed and demonstrated no synchronous disease. She underwent lumpectomy, which demonstrated a 2.4-cm invasive ductal carcinoma.

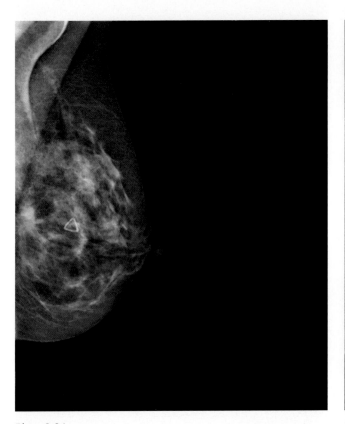

Plate 8.3A

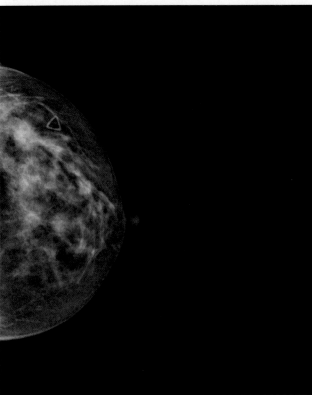

Plate 8.3B

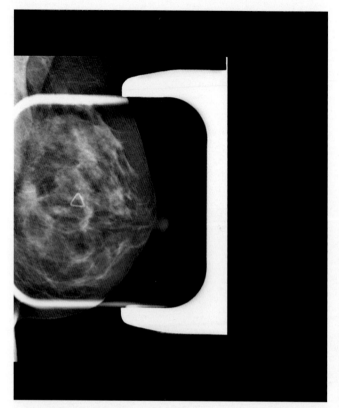

Plate 8.3C

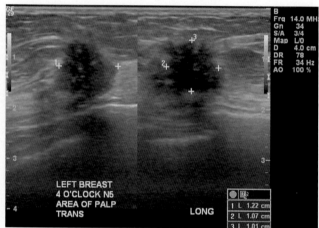

Plate 8.3D

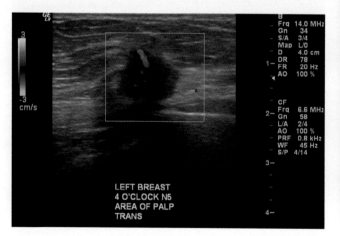

Plate 8.3E

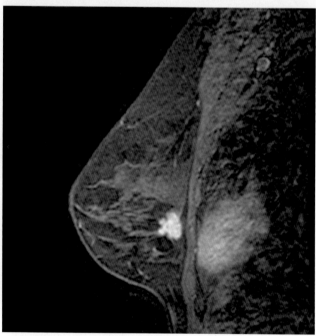

Plate 8.3F

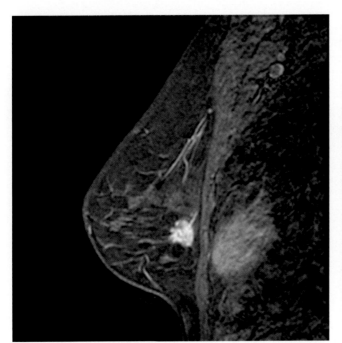

Plate 8.3G

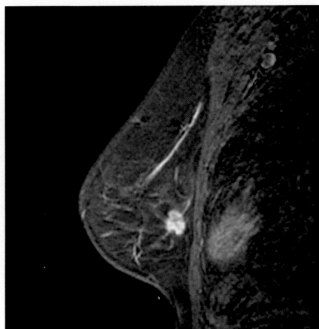

Plate 8.3H

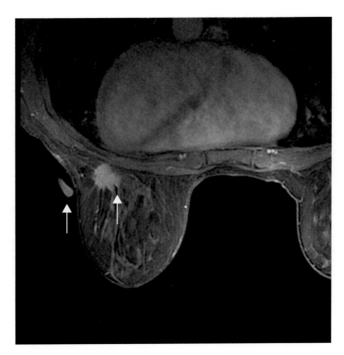

Plate 8.3I

FINDINGS

- Plates 8.3A–C—Demonstrate digital image with heterogeneous dense parenchyma and a spiculated mass posterior to the triangular marker placed over the palpable lesion.
- Plates 8.3D–E—Demonstrates a 1.2-cm hypoechoic, markedly irregular mass abutting the pectoral muscle, with shadowing and increased blood flow. The mass appears much smaller on US than on the MRI that followed.
- Plates 8.3F–H—Demonstrate a 1.8-cm irregular enhancing mass. Notice again the feeding vessel posteriorly.
- Plate 8.3I—An axial image demonstrating the vitamin E capsule over the abnormality and the subjacent enhancing mass. The spiculations become more evident on these delayed images.

• Plate 4

HISTORY

A 71-year-old woman presented with an abnormal screening breast US (performed for heterogeneously dense breasts on digital mammography). An US-guided core biopsy was performed and demonstrated the presence of apocrine-type invasive ductal carcinoma. An MRI was performed for extent of disease evaluation and demonstrated a left upper outer quadrant enhancing mass. In addition, clumped linear and nodular enhancement is noted in the left retroareolar region and the left lower breast. Subsequent US- and MRI-guided core biopsies demonstrated additional areas of invasive ductal and DCIS. She underwent mastectomy and final pathology demonstrated multicentric invasive ductal carcinoma with extensive associated DCIS and two positive axillary nodes.

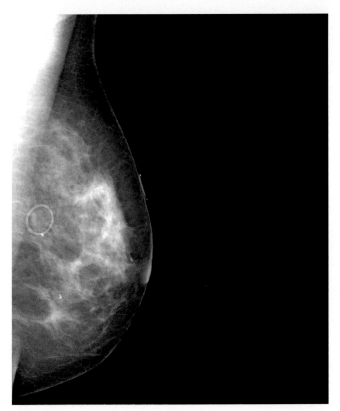

Plate 8.4A

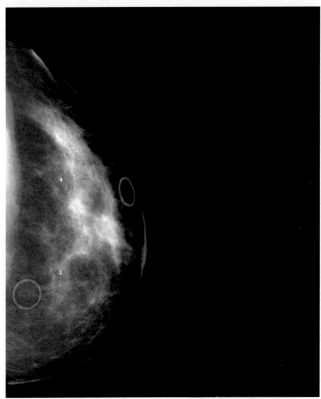

Plate 8.4B

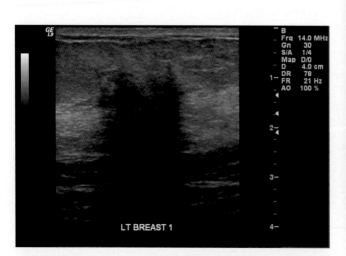

Plate 8.4C

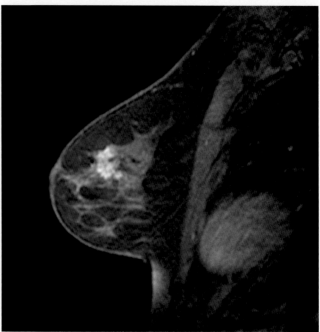

Plate 8.4D

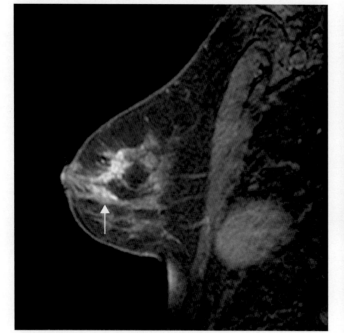

Plate 8.4E

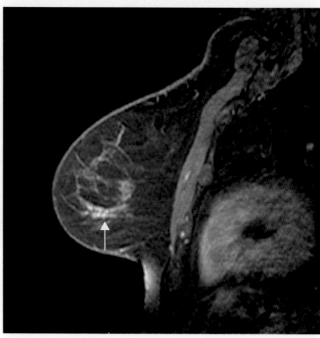

Plate 8.4F

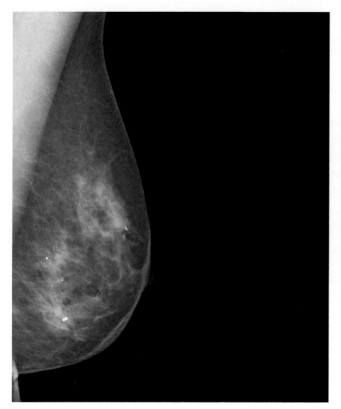

Plate 8.4G

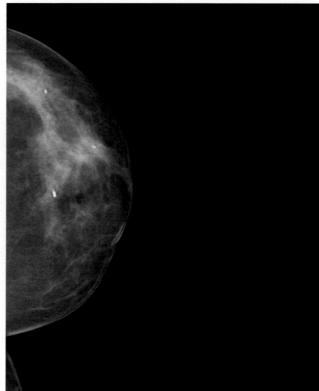

Plate 8.4H

FINDINGS

- Plates 8.4A–B—Demonstrate digital mammographic images with heterogeneous dense parenchyma with circular mole marker and a metallic clip from a remote history of prior benign core biopsy. The mammographic findings have been considered stable, but in retrospect there is a suggestion of density/distortion seen in the superareolar region on the mediolateral oblique view only.

- Plate 8.4C—Demonstrate sonographic image showing a shadowing area with irregular borders and increased vascularity, suspicious for malignancy. This was biopsied and found to represent apocrine type invasive ductal carcinoma.

- Plate 8.4D—Sagittal postcontrast image demonstrating a 2-cm irregular enhancing mass, with artifact from clip that had been placed at the time of core biopsy.

- Plates 8.4E–F—Demonstrate additional areas of suspicious enhancement in the retroareolar area and lower breast. MRI- and US-guided core biopsies of these areas were performed and demonstrated DCIS and invasive ductal carcinoma.

- Plates 8.4G–H—Postbiopsy images demonstrate the clips at multiple sites of biopsy-proven invasive and in situ carcinoma.

INVASIVE LOBULAR CARCINOMA

• CASE 1

HISTORY

A 69-year-old woman with a family history of breast cancer who presented with abnormal first high risk screening magnetic resonance imaging (MRI). She had a 1-cm clumped area of enhancement in the right upper breast in the 12:00 axis.

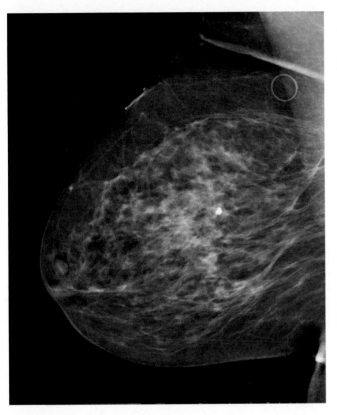

Figure 9.1A

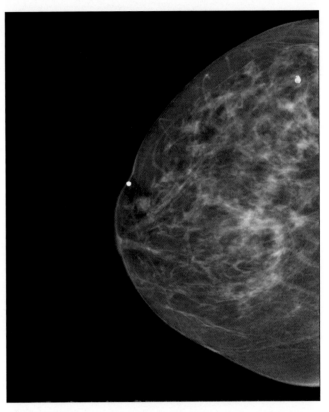

Figure 9.1B

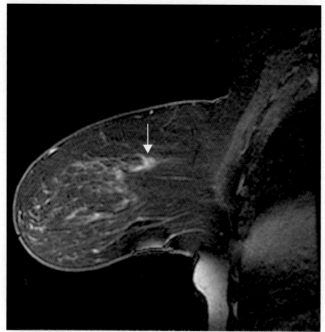

Figure 9.1C

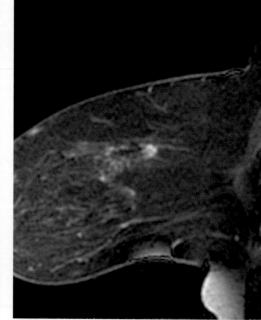

Figure 9.1D

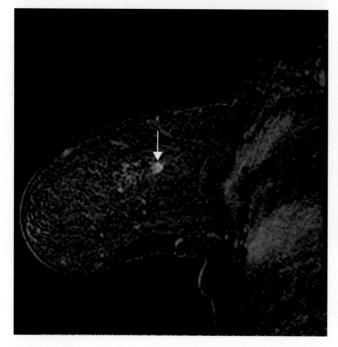

Figure 9.1E

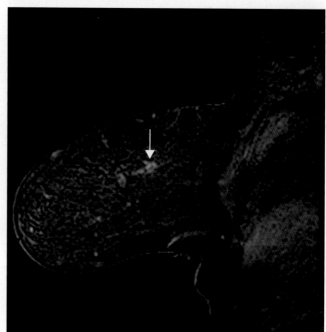

Figure 9.1F

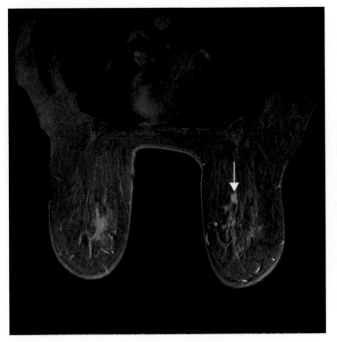

Figure 9.1G

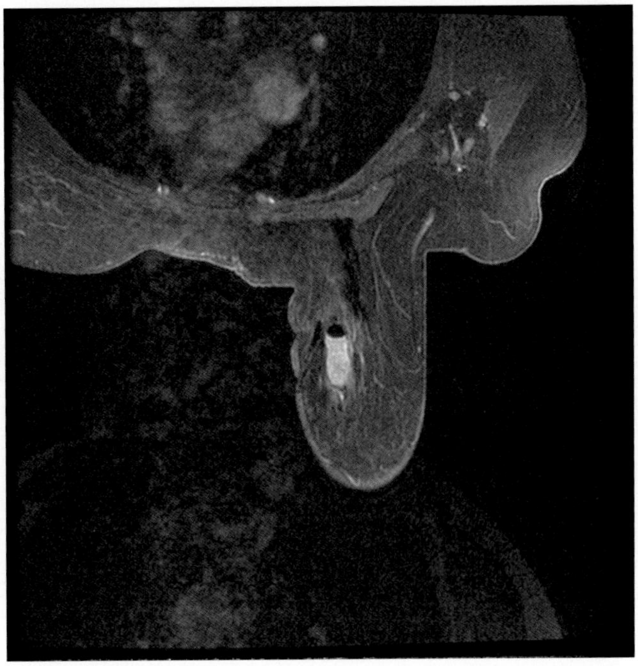

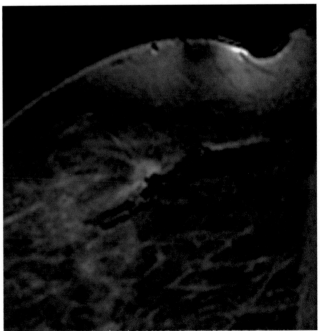

Figure 9.1H

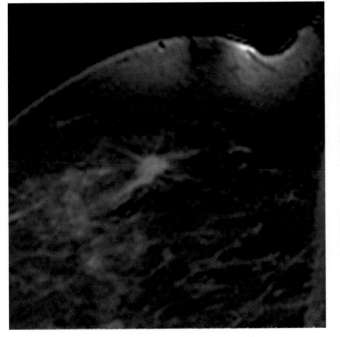

Figure 9.1I

Figure 9.1J

FINDINGS

- Figures 9.1A–B—Right mammogram demonstrating heterogeneously dense parenchyma. A palpable nodule near the nipple was found on ultrasound (US) to represent a cyst. In retrospect, in the posterior most aspect of the right breast, CC view only, there is a small soft tissue density, but this had been stable as compared with prior exams.
- Figures 9.1C–F—Sagittal post contrast and subtraction series, demonstrating an 8mm irregular faintly enhancing nodule with some minimal ring enhancement and a small amount of adjacent linear enhancement extending anteriorly.
- Figure 9.1G—Axial image demonstrating the small mass in the right breast.
- Figure 9.1H—Axial image after core biopsy demonstrating the fluid and air containing cavity at the site where the nodule was previously identified.
- Figures 9.1I–J—Magnified images of pre and post biopsy of the lesion.

WORKUP

- A targeted ultrasound of the area was negative. She underwent a MRI guided core biopsy. Pathology revealed invasive lobular carcinoma. She underwent lumpectomy with wire localization and sentinel node biopsy. Final pathology 1.1-cm invasive lobular with negative sentinel nodes.

DISCUSSION

Invasive lobular carcinomas are classically difficult to detect on digital mammography as well as clinically. MRI is more sensitive at detecting these lesions, but despite that, some of these lesions can demonstrate very subtle findings. There is also some variability in enhancement of lesions, which may limit detection. Some lobular carcinomas enhance so faintly and slowly (progressively) that they are missed on MRI. For these types of lesions, the most delayed images yield the most information about morphology. These lesions may also enhance inconsistently, being more prominent on the diagnostic than it is on the day of the biopsy (or vice versa, as in this case). The most important feature of these lesions relates to morphology; spiculation and architectural distortion are very suspicious findings. Ring enhancement is also a very suspicious finding on MRI.

This lesion was only moderately suspicious appearing on the initial MR exam. However, interpretation in conjunction with digital mammography and/or ultrasound enables the best assessment to help decide if something noted is truly suspicious. Use of all breast imaging studies helped to determine that the initial lesion seen on diagnostic MRI is quite suspicious, and the appropriate action was taken. In this case, the lesion on diagnostic MRI was somewhat suspicious, but when coupled with the retrospective findings on digital mammography, the level of suspicion increased and biopsy was promptly performed.

During MRI core biopsy, targeting should confirm that the needle is in or adjacent to the lesion. Post biopsy images should confirm that at least a portion of the lesion has been removed. We perform biopsies using sagittal images. If it is unclear on sagittal views that a portion is removed, use the axial images to see if the biopsy cavity corresponds to the expected location of the lesion.

• CASE 2

HISTORY

A 62-year-old woman who presented with nipple retraction and a palpable mass. digital Mammography demonstrated asymmetry in breast size, with the left being smaller than the right. There was nipple retractment perioareolar skin thickening with some asymmetric density in the left outer breast, but no discrete mass was seen on digital mammography. Initial ultrasound was negative.

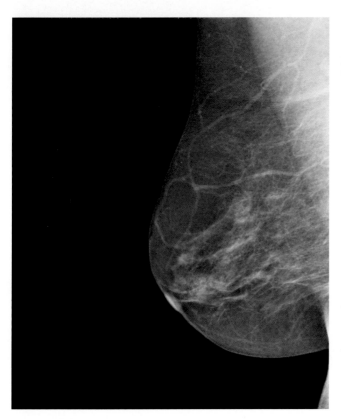

Figure 9.2A

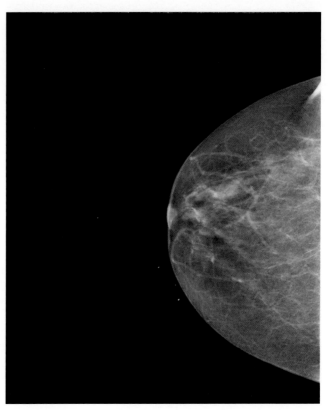

Figure 9.2B

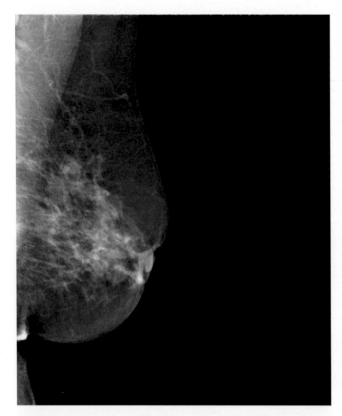

Figure 9.2C

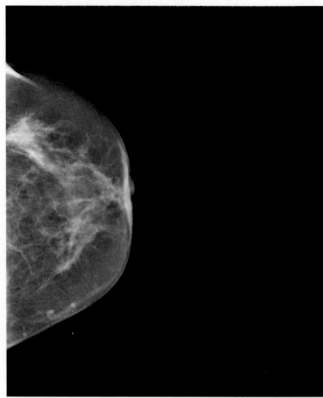

Figure 9.2D

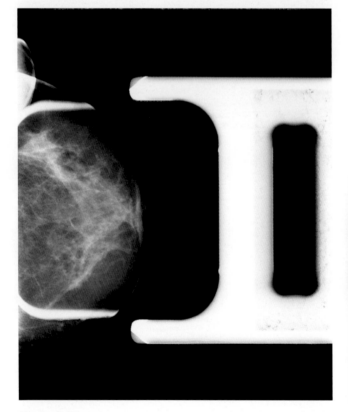

Figure 9.2E

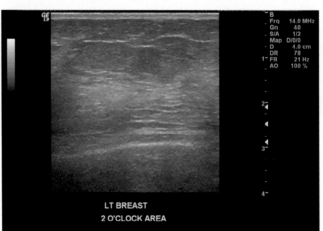

Figure 9.2F

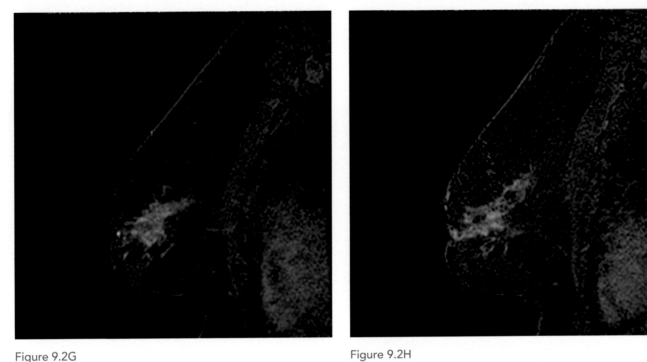

Figure 9.2G

Figure 9.2H

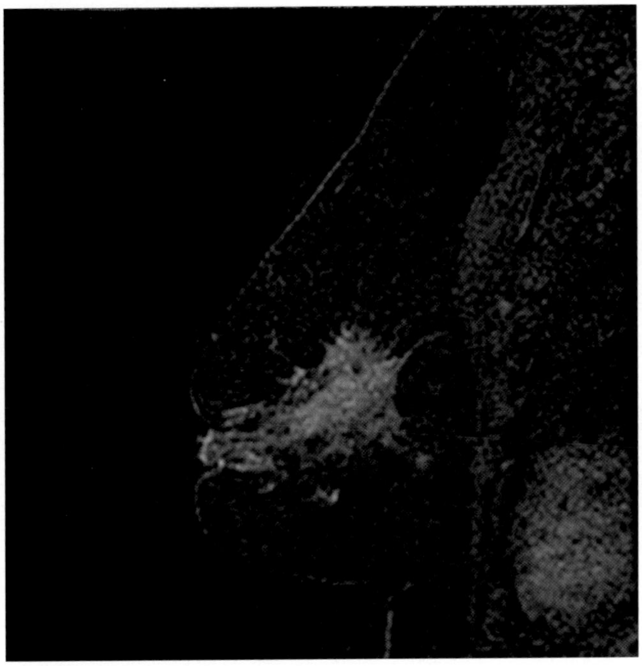

Figure 9.2I

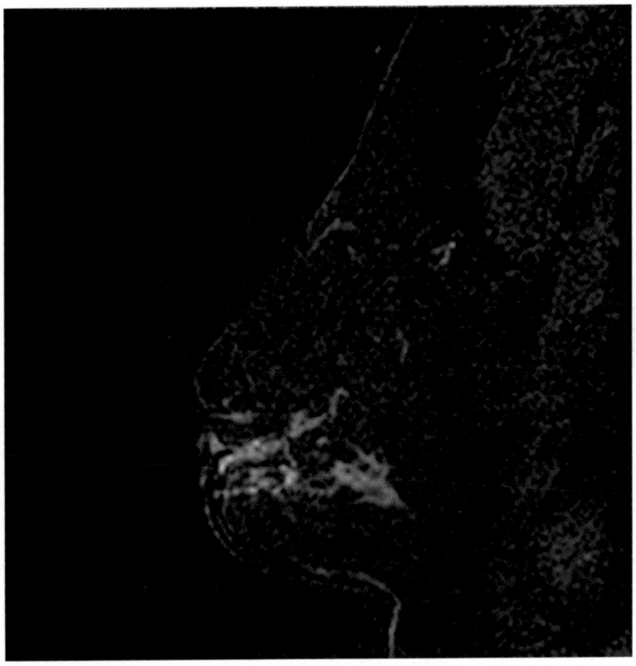

Figure 9.2J

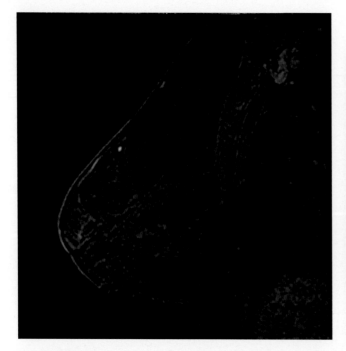

Figure 9.2K

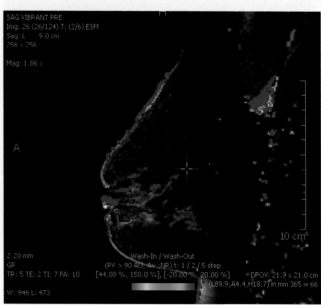

Figure 9.2L

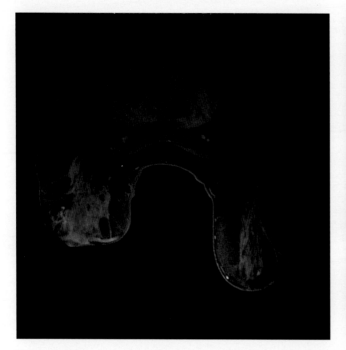

Figure 9.2M

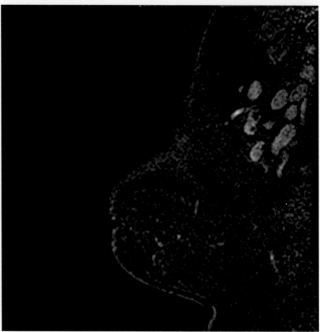

Figure 9.2N

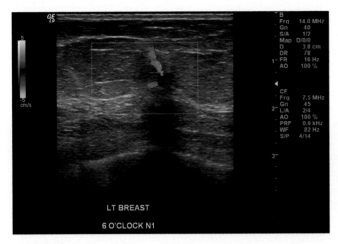

Figure 9.2O

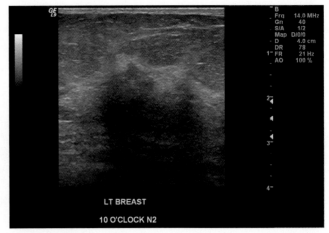

Figure 9.2P

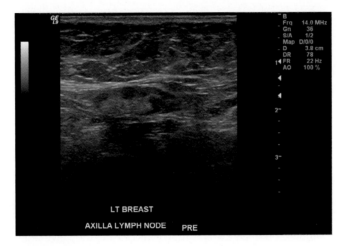

Figure 9.2Q

FINDINGS

- Figures 9.2A–B—Mammogram demonstrating normal appearing right breast with mixed fibroglandular and fatty tissue.
- Figures 9.2C–D—Demonstrate the smaller left breast with asymmetric outer soft tissue but no discrete mass. There is nipple retraction and periareolar skin thickening.
- Figure 9.2E—Compression spot view with no discrete mass.
- Figure 9.2F—Initial ultrasound of the palpable area shows no abnormality.
- Figures 9.2G–J—Subtracted sagittal images demonstrating extensive enhancement involving all four quadrants of the left breast.
- Figure 9.2K—Sagittal view of the right breast for comparison demonstrating no background glandular enhancement.
- Figure 9.2L—Color enhanced image diffuse faint progressively enhancing foci, which could be mistaken for glandular enhancement in a different setting (left breast).
- Figure 9.2M—Axial view demonstrating the marked asymmetry in size and enhancement.
- Figure 9.2N—Demonstrates a sagittal view of the left axilla with severe adenopathy.
- Figures 9.2O–P—Demonstrates targeted ultrasound, performed two weeks after initial. ultrasound, showing shadowing hypoechoic areas with increased vascularity corresponding to areas of abnormal enhancement on MRI.

- Figure 9.2Q—Sonography of an axillary lymph node with thickening of the cortex at the superior pole.

WORKUP

- MRI was performed as part of clinical problem solving. MRI demonstrated extensive (4-quadrant) left breast enhancement, linear and clumped, as well as grouped ("clustered") enhancing foci. Also seen is severe left axillary lymphadenopathy. A second-look targeted ultrasound was performed and several hypoechoic areas were identified, corresponding to areas of abnormal enhancement on MRI. Needle core biopsy of multiple areas was performed as well as fine-need aspiration of the axillary lymph node with ultrasound guidance. Pathology revealed invasive lobular carcinoma in the three areas targeted. The lymph node cytology was suspicious for metastatic carcinoma. She underwent mastectomy, which showed multicentric invasive lobular carcinoma, with the largest lesion at 7 cm, with invasion into the nipple and 33/33 lymph nodes positive for metastatic disease.

DISCUSSION

On digital mammography, the signs of invasive lobular ca can be very subtle. In this case, the entire breast is involved, but there is no discrete mass. This appearance is typical for an advanced invasive lobular carcinoma and is called the "shrinking breast" sign. The breast has retracted and increased in density, findings that are suspicious for diffuse carcinoma, especially lobular. The MRI findings are reflective of the mammographic findings in that the breast appears diminished in size as compared to the contralateral breast. The enhancement of the malignancy is more conspicuous when compared to the normal side. Knowing that the tumor involved all four quadrants, repeat targeted ultrasound was able to demonstrate multiple vague, subtle hypoechoic areas, which can be easily biopsied with sonographic guidance. Although we do not recommend targeted ultrasound for small solitary lesions (less than or equal to 1 cm), it is very useful for diffuse carcinoma, as multiple biopsies are more easily performed with sonographic guidance than MRI guidance.

On some of the images, the appearance of the left breast enhancement is so diffuse that it could be confused with glandular enhancement. The marked asymmetry to the other side should alert you to this being outside the range of normal of glandular enhancement. Other findings that help alert you are areas of distortion, corresponding mammographic and clinical findings, and of course, obvious axillary adenopathy.

Obvious axillary adenopathy seen on MRI should be evaluated with an ultrasound-guided biopsy of abnormal appearing lymph nodes. Confirming the presence of axillary involvement prior to surgery will obviate the need for sentinel node biopsy, and the surgeon can proceed directly to axillary dissection. Metastatic lobular carcinoma is much more difficult for the pathologist to diagnose on cytology, and although fine-needle aspiration biopsy of axillary nodes works well for metastatic ductal carcinoma, core biopsy may be necessary to confirm metastatic lobular carcinoma.

• CASE 3

HISTORY

51-year-old woman presents with an abnormal screening mammogram, which demonstrated a 1-cm asymmetric density seen on the craniocaudal (CC) view only. Targeted US was performed and was negative.

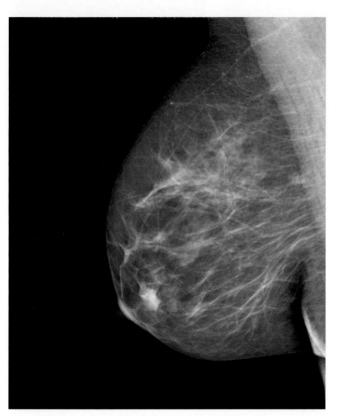

Figure 9.3A

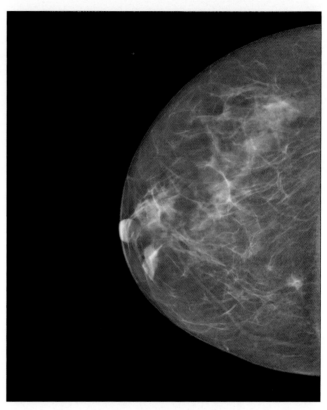

Figure 9.3B

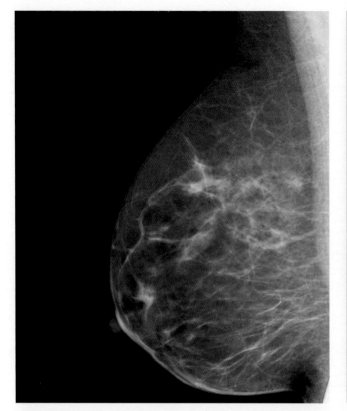

Figure 9.3C

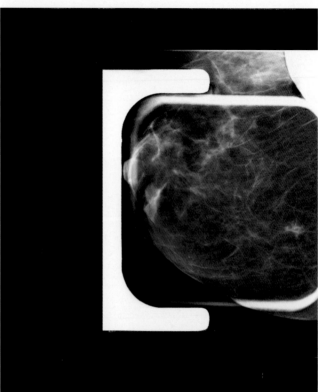

Figure 9.3D

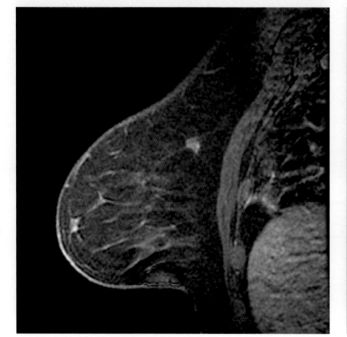

Figure 9.3E

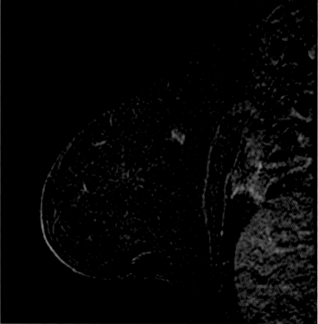

Figure 9.3F

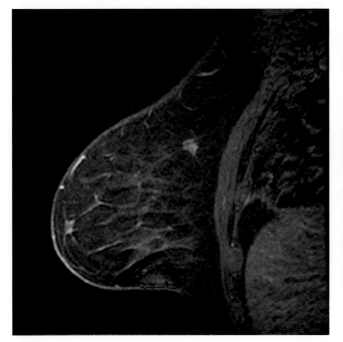

Figure 9.3G

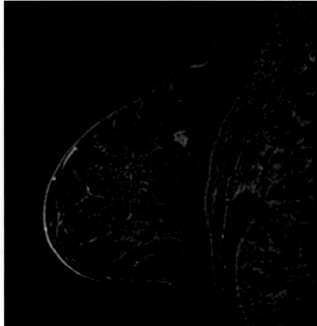

Figure 9.3H

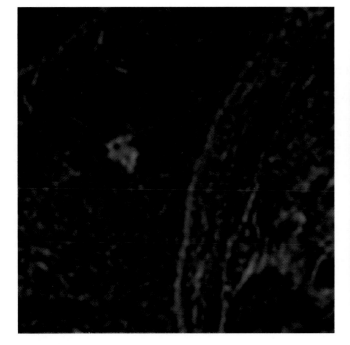

Figure 9.3I

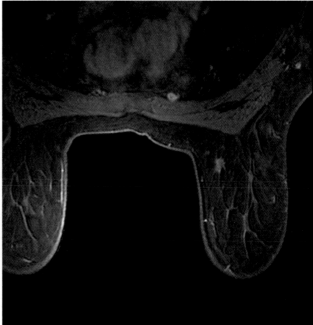

Figure 9.3J

FINDINGS

- Figures 9.3A–D—Digital mammographic images demonstrating fatty breasts with an asymmetric density in the right inner breast, which was new compared to previous exams, not definitively seen on perpendicular (mediolateral oblique, mediolateral) views.
- Figures 9.3E–F—First postcontrast and first subtracted series demonstrating faint ring enhancement in an irregular nodule in the right upper inner posterior breast.
- Figure 9.3G—Fourth postcontrast series. Because this enhancement is relatively subtle, the findings are more obvious on subtracted series.
- Figures 9.3H–I—Fourth subtracted series. More delayed images demonstrate more intense enhancement with more spiculation of the margin and more obvious ring enhancement. These findings are very suspicious for malignancy. Figure 9.3I is a magnified view.
- Figure 9.3J—Delayed axial series. Demonstrates a spiculated enhancing mass. Because this lesion enhanced progressively, it is well visualized on the delayed series.

WORKUP

- MRI was performed for problem solving ('one view only' finding). The MRI demonstrated a spiculated 1-cm faintly enhancing nodule in the area of concern. A stereotactic biopsy was performed and pathology revealed an invasive lobular carcinoma. She underwent lumpectomy, which yielded a 1.2-cm carcinoma with negative margins but two sentinel nodes were noted to be positive. An axillary dissection was performed demonstrating four positive lymph nodes.

DISCUSSION

This is a relatively classic presentation of an invasive lobular carcinoma. They can be very subtle or even undetectable on digital mammography, especially in dense breasted woman or within glandular areas of normal density breasts (e.g., retroareolar or upper outer quadrant regions where there tends to be more glandular tissue). The majority enhance on MRI: some can be less conspicuous, but fortunately very few are completely non-enhancing on MRI. When the breast parenchyma is fatty, US is less helpful. MRI is not only helpful for diagnosis, but can also be helpful with planning for core biopsy or localization for excisional biopsy. Unfortunately, even though this lesion is quite small, the patient did already have nodal metastasis.

• CASE 4

HISTORY

A 46-year-old woman who had been undergoing annual screening digital mammography but presented with the interval development of a new left upper outer quadrant palpable mass, which was found to correspond to a new 1.2-cm nodule on digital mammography and sonography.

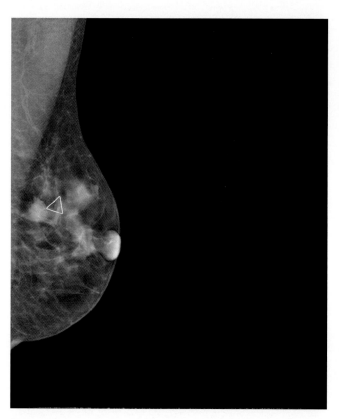

Figure 9.4A

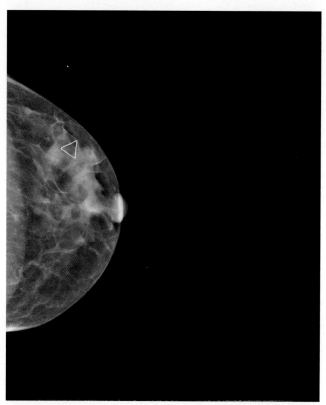

Figure 9.4B

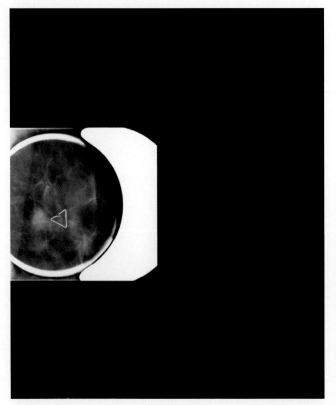

Figure 9.4C

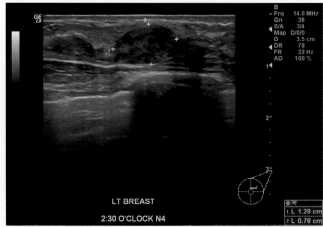

Figure 9.4D

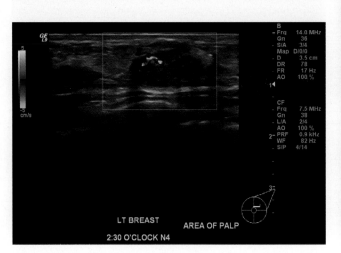

Figure 9.4E

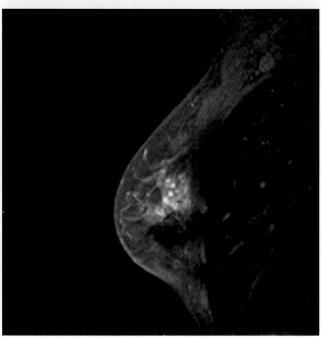

Figure 9.4F

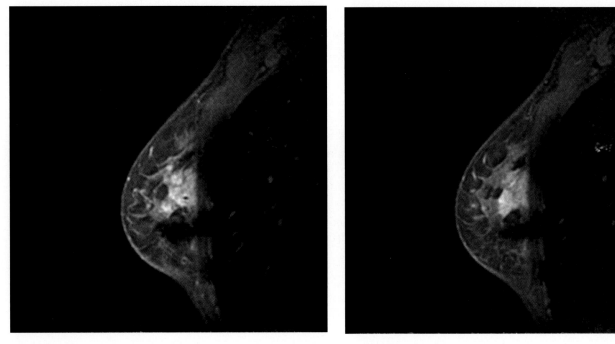

Figure 9.4G

Figure 9.4H

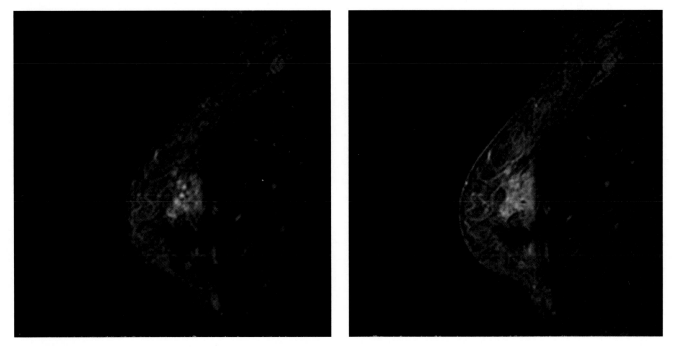

Figure 9.4I

Figure 9.4J

FINDINGS

- Figures 9.4A–C—Digital mammographic images of the left breast with mixed fibroglandular/fatty tissues and a 1.2-cm rounded nodule with indistinct margins in the upper outer quadrant, posterior aspect, corresponding to the palpable nodule.
- Figures 9.4D–E—US Demonstrating a corresponding ovoid hypoechoic solid nodule with increased internal vascularity, relatively sharply defined margins, heterogeneous internal echogenicity, measuring approximately 1.2 cm.
- Figures 9.4F–H—First, intermediate, and last postcontrast series. First postcontrast series demonstrates multiple grouped ("clustered") enhancing foci, spanning a 3.5-cm area in the left upper outer quadrant posteriorly, corresponding to the area of palpable abnormality, but appearing larger than was noted clinically and mammographically/sonographically.
- Figures 9.4I–J—First and last subtracted image. The subtracted images demonstrate the same findings, but as usual makes them more conspicuous.

WORKUP

- This nodule was biopsied using sonographic guidance. Final pathology demonstrated invasive lobular carcinoma on core biopsy. The MRI was done for extent of disease evaluation. The area of suspicious enhancement extended 3.5 cm, considered larger than was suspected. The patient opted for bilateral mastectomies (personal preference). Final pathology revealed a 4-cm invasive lobular carcinoma with multiple positive lymph nodes.

DISCUSSION

Invasive lobular carcinoma can be subtle to diagnose even on MRI. These lesions may not present as a discrete mass, but rather as grouped enhancing foci. We refer to this appearance as a "cluster" of enhancing foci. Because invasive lobulars can have progressive enhancement kinetics, the size and margins of the lesion can sometimes be better appreciated on the more delayed contrast series. On the more delayed images, you can see the filling in between the enhancing foci and appreciate the relatively large area of the enhancement. Usually the size of the lesion is more accurately assessed on MRI then on mammogram or US. The more superior accuracy of measuring size is the reason MRI is the modality of choice for measuring response to neoadjuvant chemotherapy.

However, even MRI can over or under predict the size of the lesion. Underestimation of tumor size can occur for several reasons. Some cancers have microscopic extensions or scattered rests of cells that cannot be detected because of small (microscopic) size. Also, some areas may contain macroscopic tumor, but for other reasons (e.g., compression, postchemotherapy fibrosis) fail to enhance. Conversely, surrounding glandular or fibrocystic enhancement, or postbiopsy inflammation/enhancement, may mimic disease extension and overestimate tumor size.

• CASE 5

HISTORY

A 66-year-old woman presents with an outside mammogram demonstrating left 3:00 breast axis (posteriorly) increased calcifications, for which biopsy was recommended. Stereotactic biopsy demonstrated atypical ductal hyperplasia (ADH).

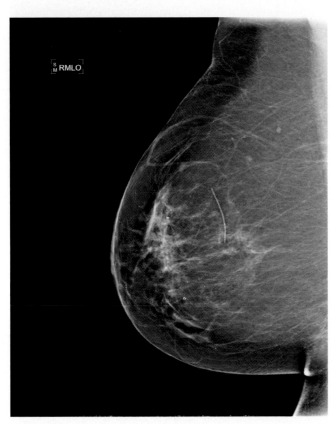

Figure 9.5A

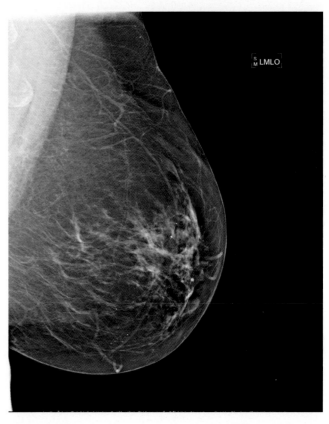

Figure 9.5B

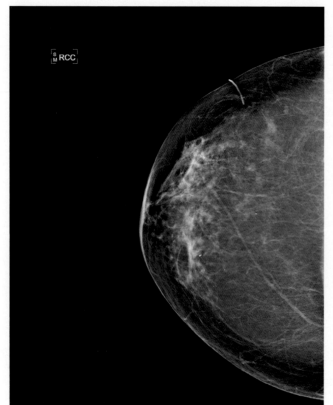

Figure 9.5C

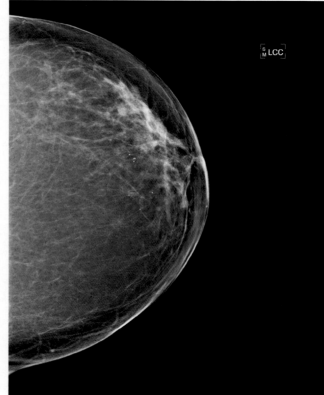

Figure 9.5D

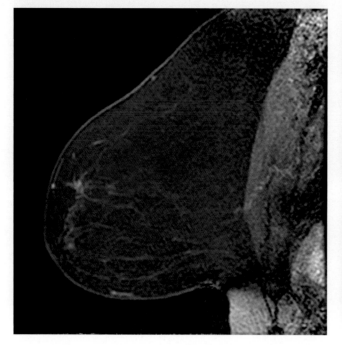

Figure 9.5E

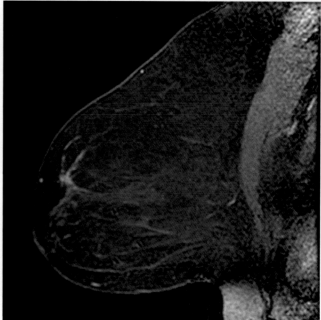

Figure 9.5F

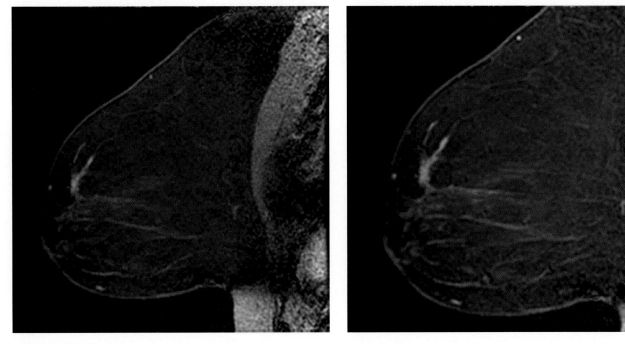

Figure 9.5G

Figure 9.5H

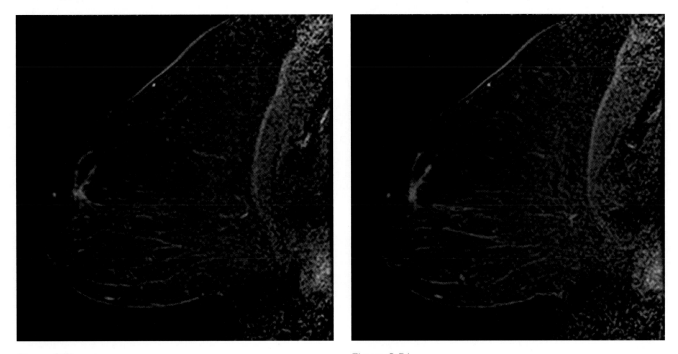

Figure 9.5I

Figure 9.5J

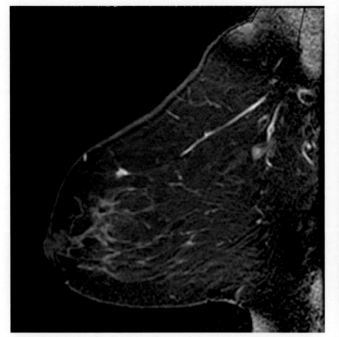

Figure 9.5K

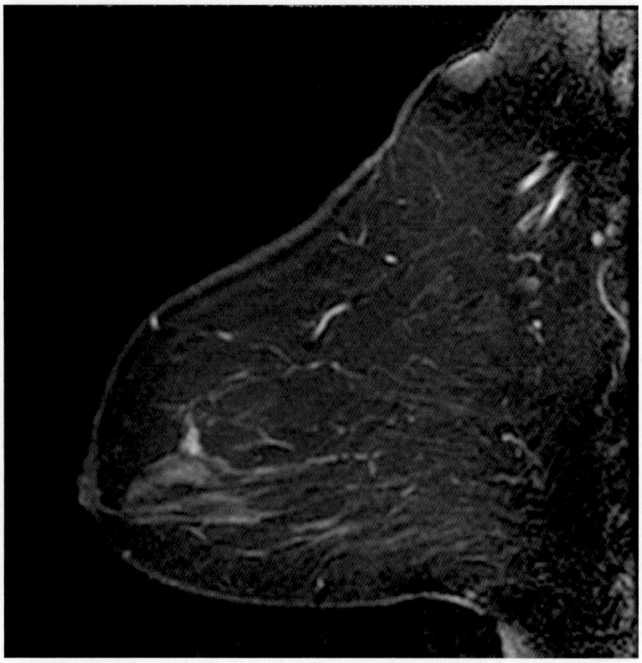

Figure 9.5L

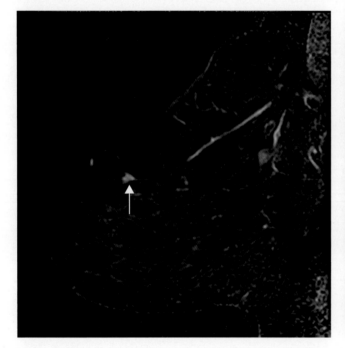

Figure 9.5M

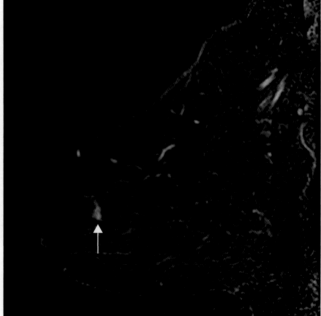

Figure 9.5N

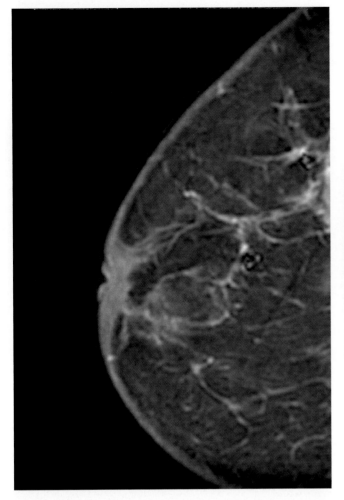

Figure 9.5O

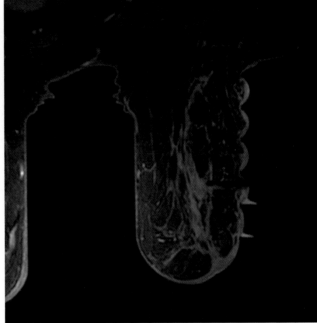

Figure 9.5P

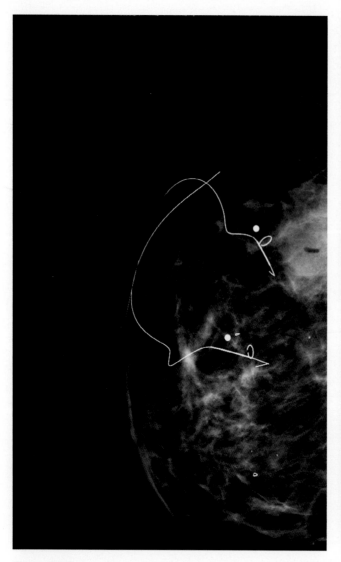

Figure 9.5Q

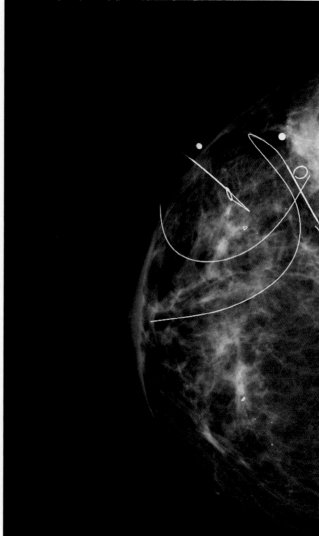

Figure 9.5R

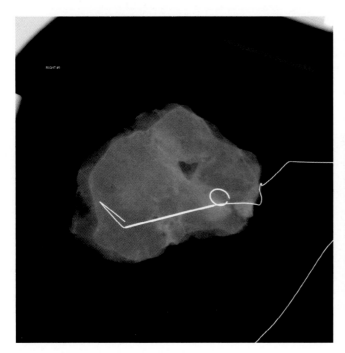

Figure 9.5S

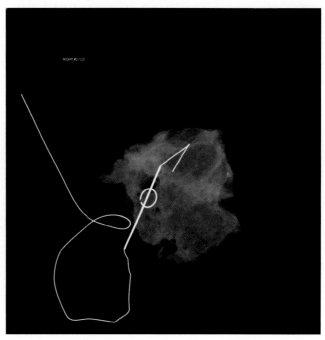

Figure 9.5T

FINDINGS

- Figures 9.5A–D—Digital mammographic images demonstrating bilateral scattered and grouped calcifications. The right breast has a metallic clip from a previous benign needle biopsy, as well as postsurgical changes from a previous benign excisional biopsy. The breast parenchyma is fatty.
- Figures 9.5E–H—Left postcontrast series.
- Figures 9.5I–J—Left subtracted series demonstrating a spiculated, faintly enhancing left supra areolar nodule with an associated irregular linear enhancement. No abnormal enhancement was seen at the stereotactic biopsy site, in the 3:00 axis, posteriorly.
- Figures 9.5K–L—Right postcontrast series.
- Figures 9.5M–N—Right subtraction series demonstrates two small irregular enhancing right upper outer quadrant nodules (arrow).
- Figures 9.5O–P—Sagittal and axial images from right breast MRI-guided needle localization.
- Figures 9.5Q–R—CC of lateral views from mammogram immediately post-MRI localization. Circular clips are noted. We use these to identify MRI-guided localization sites, for the infrequent cases in which prior core biopsy/clip placement has not been previously performed.
- Figures 9.5S–T—Specimen radiographs demonstrating and confirming successful excision of localized MRI abnormalities.

WORKUP

- Stereotactic core biopsy of left outer posterior 3:00 axis calcifications had demonstrated atypical hyperplasia. She underwent excisional biopsy, which was preceded by MRI because of her elevated risk status. The preoperative MRI demonstrated an irregular suspicious left-enhancing mass and associated linear enhancement in the 12:00 axis anteriorly, as well as two smaller suspicious irregular enhancing nodules in the *right* upper outer quadrant. Additional bilateral core biopsies were recommended. The left breast core biopsy demonstrated ductal carcinoma in situ. Attempted core biopsy of the right breast was complicated by hematoma and therefore surgical excisional right breast biopsy was performed at the time of left breast lumpectomy. Final pathology demonstrated a left breast 12:00 axis 0.9-cm invasive ductal carcinoma with associated solid and comedo type extensive intraductal component. The right upper outer quadrant demonstrated two foci (0.2 and 0.7 cm) of invasive lobular carcinoma. Bilateral sentinel node biopsies were negative. Excisional biopsy of the original area of concern (left outer) demonstrated only ADH.

DISCUSSION

This is a very interesting and complicated case that began as a routine screening mammogram with slightly suspicious findings of increased calcifications, in a patient with multiple previous benign biopsies and numerous areas of calcifications in both breasts. Even though the patient has fatty breasts, there is no mammographic abnormality to be seen at the site of her left breast supraareolar invasive ductal carcinoma/ductal carcinoma in situ or at the site of multifocal invasive lobular in the right upper outer quadrant. In this case, if she had not had her preoperative MRI, the malignancies probably would have remained clinically occult for at least a year or more. Before the surgery date, it is important to try to sample all lesions that are significantly suspicious to better plan surgery. However, some patients are reluctant to undergo several biopsies. A nurse navigator can greatly assist the patient in making these decisions. On the rare occasion when preoperative sampling is not able to be done, a circular MRI clip is placed at the time of MRI-guided localization, to help confirm intraoperatively that the correct area is excised. Without clip placement, the radiologist and surgeon have no ability to confirm excision of an MRI abnormality. Even if you are confident of your localization wire placement, it can migrate before or during surgery, and we have seen cases where an MRI localized abnormality excised without clip confirmation of excision was still present in the breast on follow-up postexcision MRI!

Incidentally, the pathologist revealed that the 3:00 left breast calcifications that started the entire workup were completely benign, and not associated with any of the malignant or atypical areas.

● CASE 6

HISTORY

A 55-year-old woman who presented with an area of architectural distortion in the right upper outer quadrant on screening mammogram.

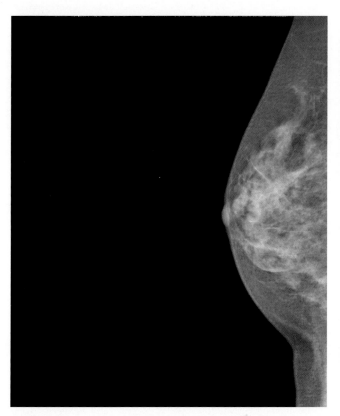

Figure 9.6A

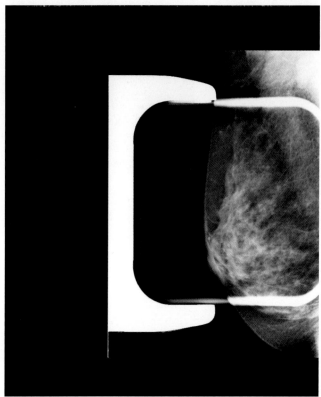

Figure 9.6B

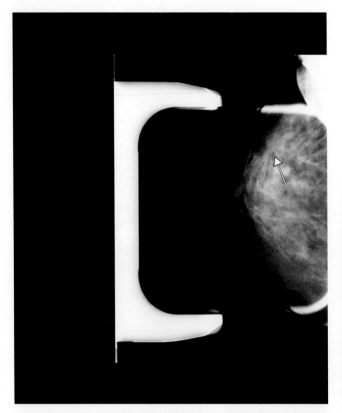

Figure 9.6C

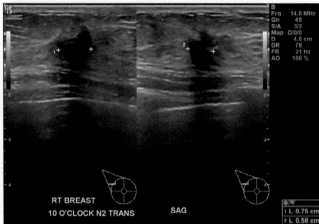

Figure 9.6D

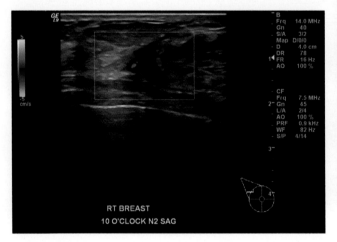

Figure 9.6E

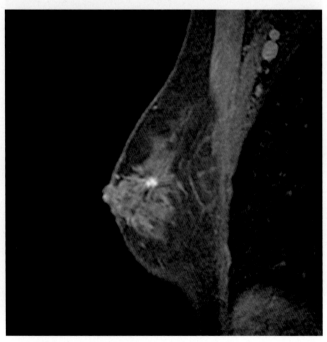

Figure 9.6F

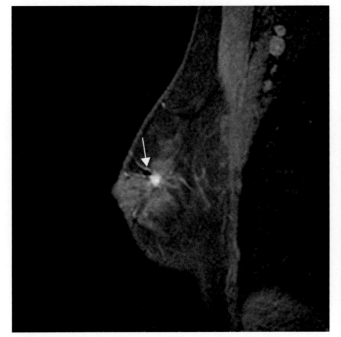

Figure 9.6G

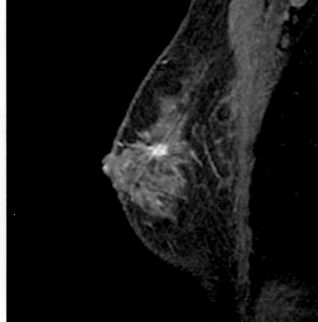

Figure 9.6H

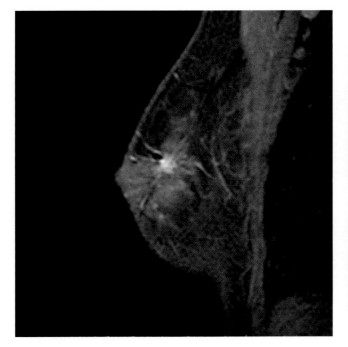

Figure 9.6I

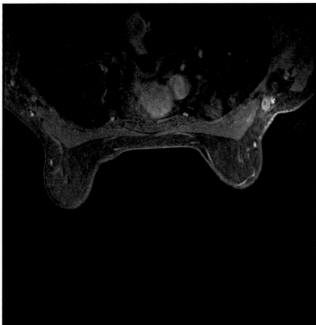

Figure 9.6J

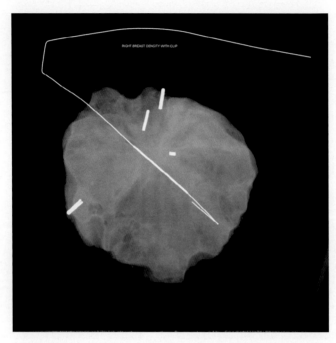

Figure 9.6K

FINDINGS

- Figures 9.6A–C—Digital mammogram images with heterogeneous dense parenchyma with subtle architectural distortion in the right upper outer quadrant, (arrow).

- Figures 9.6D–E—Demonstrates an irregular, hypoechoic, spiculated shadowing lesion with increased internal vascularity.

- Figures 9.6F–I—Sagittal postcontrast series with a small irregular enhancing nodule that appears to "blossom" on delayed images (H,I). The metallic clip is noted.

- Figure 9.6J—Axial delayed image with right axillary adenopathy demonstrated.

- Figure 9.6K—Specimen-magnified radiograph with the spiculated lesion in the central aspect, containing the clip that had been placed at US-guided core biopsy.

WORKUP

- US demonstrated a corresponding suspicious lesion, which was evaluated with needle biopsy and found to be a subcentimeter invasive lobular carcinoma. MRI scan was done as an extent of disease evaluation and demonstrated no additional suspicious lesion except for possible axillary adenopathy. Axillary fine-needle aspiration biopsy was inconclusive. She underwent lumpectomy with sentinel node biopsy. Final pathology demonstrated 0.9-cm invasive lobular with associated lobular carcinoma in situ (LCIS) and 9/13 positive lymph nodes.

DISCUSSION

Although this lesion is very subtle on digital mammography (as is not uncommon for lobular carcinomas) it is easily seen on MRI.

Fine-needle aspiration biopsy of axillary nodes is not as reliable for metastatic invasive lobular carcinoma as it is for invasive ductal, and therefore consider core biopsy of any abnormal appearing lymph nodes. A definitive diagnosis of axillary metastases before surgery will obviate the need for sentinel node biopsy, and the surgeon can perform the full axillary dissection at the same time as the lumpectomy, therefore obviating a second trip to the operating room. This case also demonstrates a not uncommon scenario of a very small primary invasive lobular carcinoma with extensive axillary involvement already present at the time of diagnosis.

• Plate 1

HISTORY

A 69-year-old woman presented with a one-view-only finding on digital mammography of an asymmetric density in left inner breast. The patient indicated to the technologist that this corresponded to an excisional benign biopsy site/scar tissue. US demonstrated a corresponding finding but was initially interpreted as also possibly representing scar tissue.

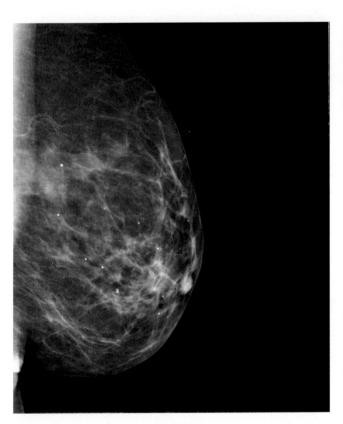

Plate 9.1A

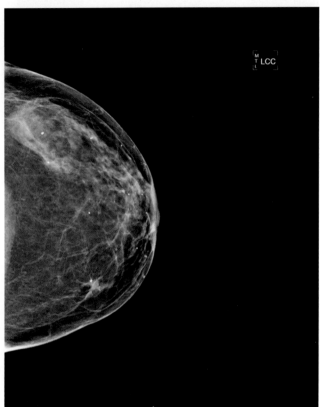

Plate 9.1B

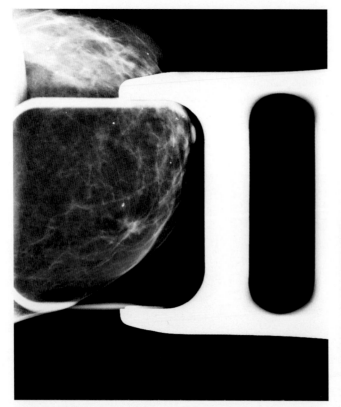

Plate 9.1C

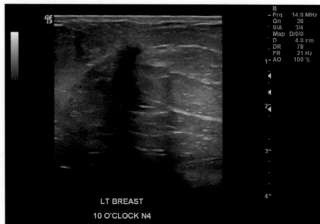

Plate 9.1D

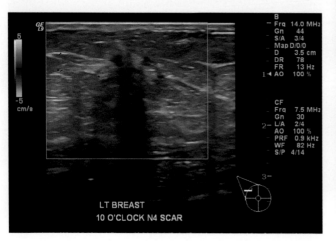

Plate 9.1E

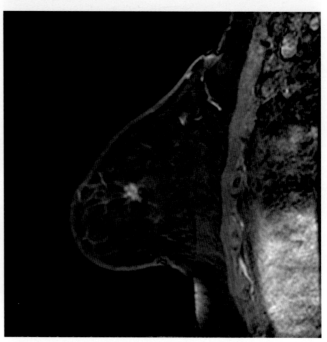

Plate 9.1F

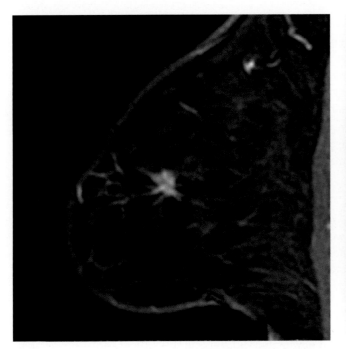

Plate 9.1G

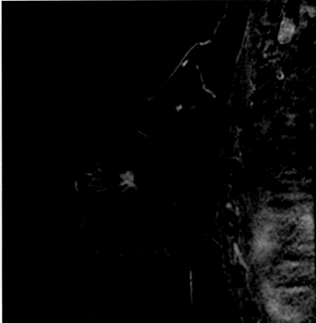

Plate 9.1H

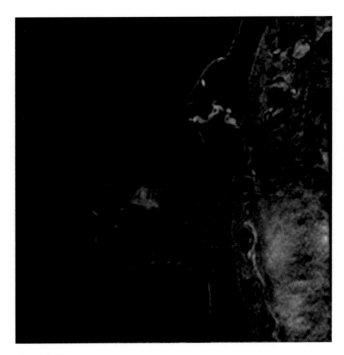

Plate 9.1I

FINDINGS

- Plates 9.1A–C—Digital mammogram demonstrating an asymmetric density in the left inner breast on one view only (CC view).
- Plates 9.1D–E—US demonstrated a hypoechoic shadowing region. In retrospect, it has a malignant appearance. However, it was initially misinterpreted as possibly represented as scar tissue, as the patient indicated that it had been present previously.
- Plates 9.1F–I—MRI scans demonstrating an obvious spiculated mass measuring 1.5 cm on initial views, highly suspicious for carcinoma. On the delayed views (I), the area "blossomed" to approximately 2 cm.

WORKUP

- MRI was recommended for mammographic problem solving ('one view only' finding). Biopsy was performed with US guidance and demonstrated invasive lobular carcinoma. She underwent lumpectomy with sentinel node biopsy; final pathology demonstrated a 3-cm invasive lobular carcinoma with negative sentinel lymph node biopsy.

DISCUSSION

One of the earliest applications of MRI was to differentiate scar from malignancy. In this case, it is clearly demonstrated how useful MRI still is in this setting. The mammographic and sonographic findings can mimic scar tissue, and when combined with the patient's insistent history of an old scar at this site, the radiologist can be misled. MRI correlation ensured that the correct diagnosis was made.

Invasive lobular can appear significantly larger on delayed images, and are frequently found to be larger at excision than they appear on mammogram, US, or MRI. Presumably, this may be related to the histology of the disease, because invasive lobular carcinoma is known for its tendency to infiltrate into the surrounding breast tissue with "Indian file" or "single rows" of tumor cells. These linear one-cell-thick cancerous extensions can be too small (microscopic) to be seen on any imaging modality, particularly when there is little host response to the disease.

• Plate 2

HISTORY

An 85-year-old woman presented with a developing density on digital mammography in the posterior aspect of the right upper outer quadrant. This persists on compression spot views and was found to correspond to hypoechoic area on ultrasound. MRI demonstrated a corresponding 2-cm spiculated enhancing mass. Biopsy was performed with sonographic guidance, and demonstrated invasive lobular carcinoma. Lumpectomy demonstrated a 2-cm invasive lobular carcinoma.

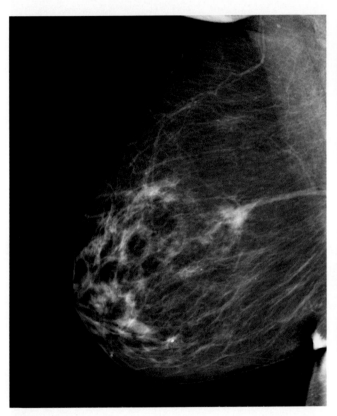

Plate 9.2A

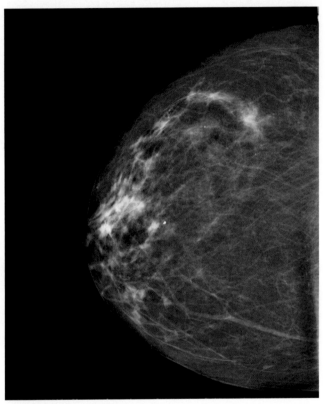

Plate 9.2B

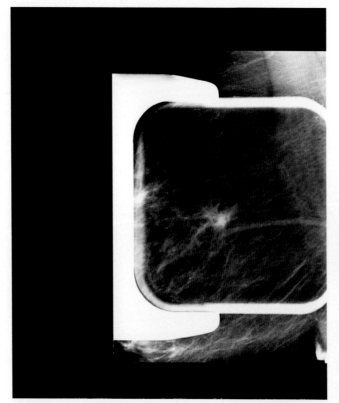

Plate 9.2C

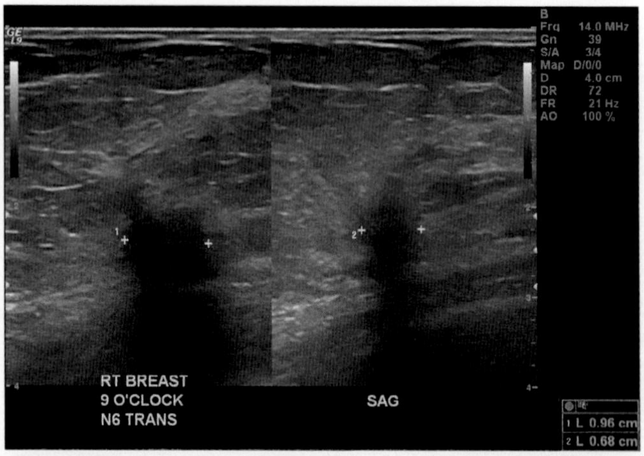

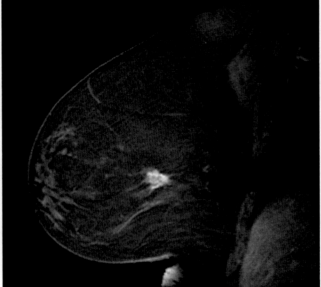

Plate 9.2D

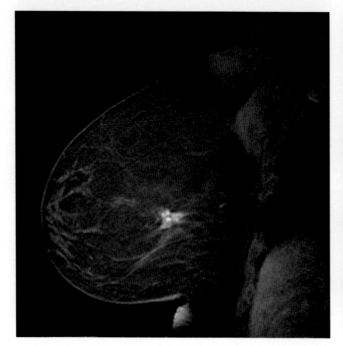

Plate 9.2E

Plate 9.2F

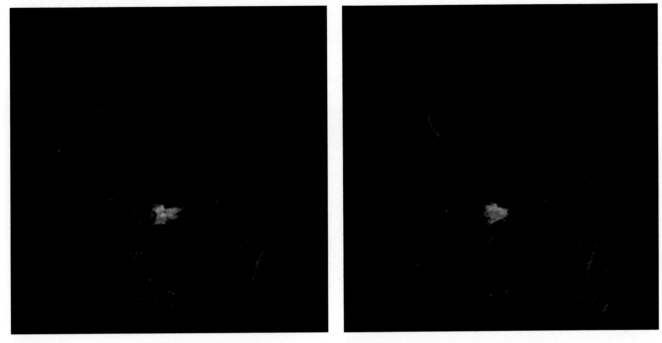

Plate 9.2G   Plate 9.2H

FINDINGS

- Plates 9.2A–C—Digital mammogram demonstrating the asymmetric, slightly spiculated density, which was not present on previous exams.
- Plate 9.2D—US images—a hypoechoic shadowing mass is demonstrated.
- Plates 9.2E–H—MRI demonstrated a spiculated enhancing mass on postcontrast and subtraction series, which "blossoms" slightly in size on more delayed images (F, H).

DISCUSSION

This is a classic presentation of an invasive lobular carcinoma. If the patient had dense breasts, the mammographic lesion may not have been detected. The availability of negative previous mammograms also made this a relatively straightforward diagnosis.

• Plate 3

HISTORY

A 57-year-old woman with a palpable right breast mass with marked deformity and "shrinkage" of the overall breast. A core biopsy was performed via US guidance, which demonstrated invasive lobular carcinoma.

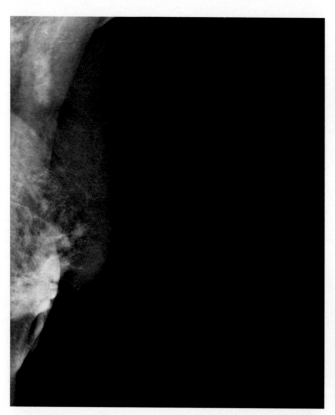

Plate 9.3A

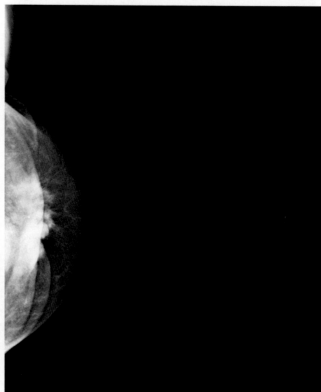

Plate 9.3B

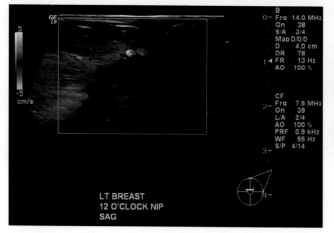

Plate 9.3C

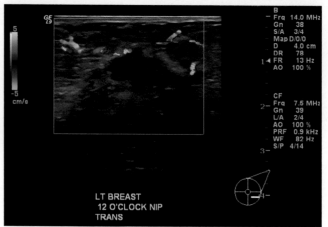

Plate 9.3D

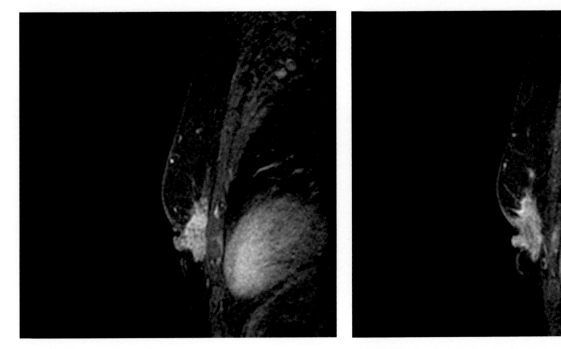

Plate 9.3E

Plate 9.3F

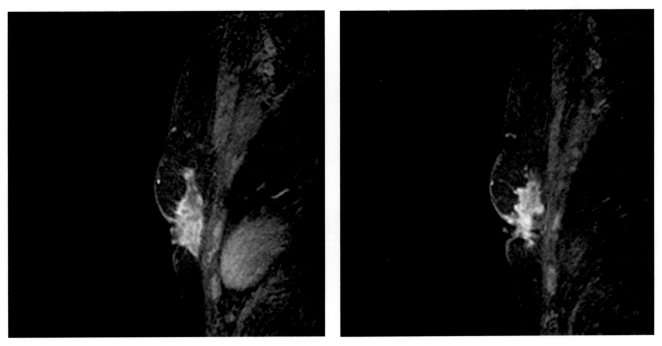

Plate 9.3G

Plate 9.3H

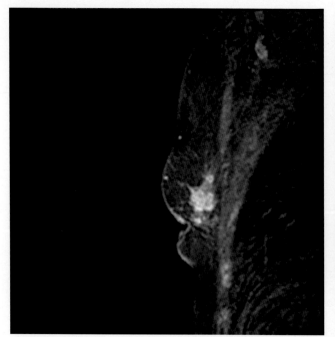

Plate 9.3I

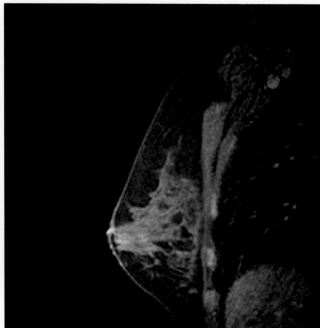

Plate 9.3J

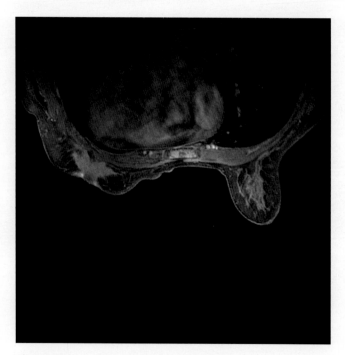

Plate 9.3K

FINDINGS

- Plates 9.3A–B—Digital mammographic views demonstrating marked deformity with inversion of the nipple and contraction of the breast.
- Plates 9.3C–D—Demonstrating large hypoechoic shadowing areas with increased vascularity.
- Plates 9.3E–I—Demonstrate extensive enhancement throughout the left breast with extension to the nipple, markedly asymmetric in size and amount of enhancement compared with the normal glandular right breast (see J).
- Plate 9.3J—Compare the abnormal left with the normal right side.
- Plate 9.3K—Axial image demonstrates marked asymmetry.

DISCUSSION

This is an unfortunate case of a large neglected invasive lobular carcinoma. When this type of carcinoma becomes very large, the enhancement may be so diffuse that it may mimic glandular enhancement and be difficult to diagnose. In this case, the marked deformity of the breast and the nipple retraction, as well as the contrast with the other normal side, makes the diagnosis much more obvious. This patient is presently undergoing neoadjuvant chemotherapy.

• **Plate 4**

HISTORY

A 59-year-old woman presented with a suspicious palpable mass. She underwent mammogram, which was negative, followed by US, which demonstrated a large heterogeneous hypoechoic 3:00 axis mass. Core biopsy was positive for invasive lobular carcinoma. She underwent MRI for extent of disease. Extensive synchronous disease was suspected and subsequent additional biopsy was performed in the 6:00 and 10:00 axes. These biopsies were also positive, confirming multicentric disease. She underwent mastectomy with sentinel node biopsy. The final pathology demonstrated multiple invasive lobular lesions, ranging in size up to 3.5 cm, as well as a positive sentinel node. Subsequent full axillary dissection demonstrated 6/13 positive nodes.

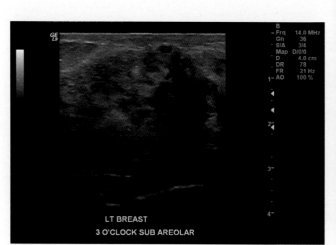

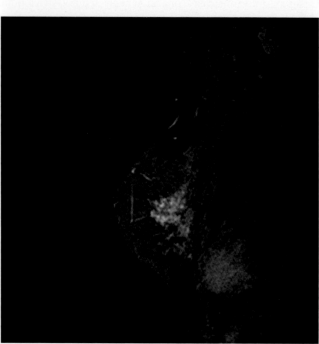

Plate 9.4A

Plate 9.4B

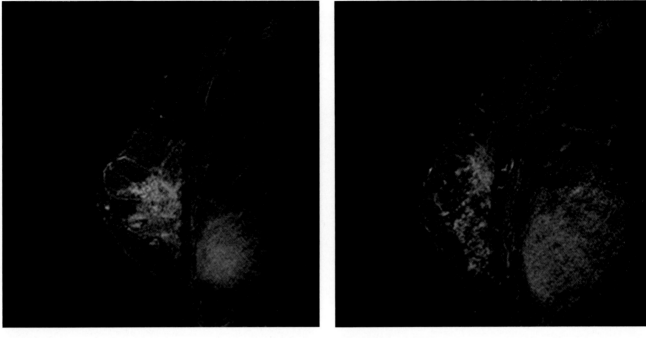

Plate 9.4C

Plate 9.4D

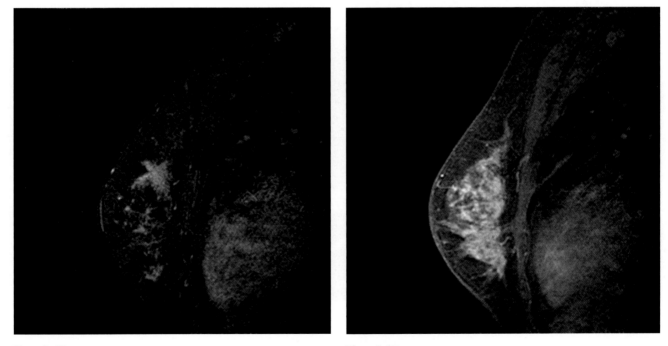

Plate 9.4E

Plate 9.4F

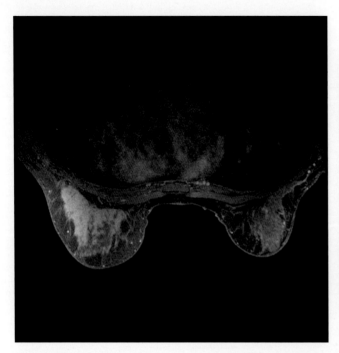

Plate 9.4G

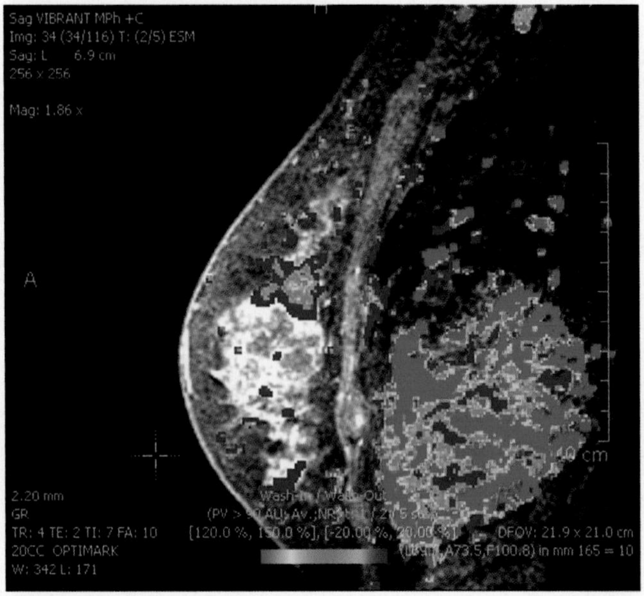

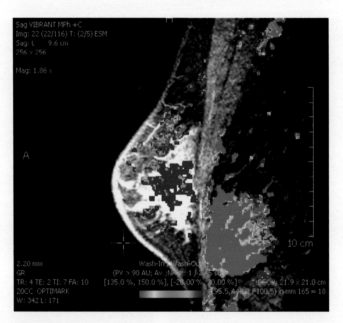

Plate 9.4H

Plate 9.4I

FINDINGS

- Plate 9.4A—US demonstrating non specific hypoechoic zones in the initial area of palpable abnormality (3:00).

- Plates 9.4B–E—Subtracted series demonstrating grouped enhancing foci and clumped/nodular enhancement in the inner upper quadrant, upper outer and lower outer quadrants.

- Plate 9.4F—More delayed postcontrast sagittal image demonstrating diffuse enhancement throughout the breast.

- Plate 9.4G—An axial view demonstrating the marked asymmetry of enhancement between the tumor replaced left breast and the normal right breast.

- Plate 9.4H—The color analysis of enhancement kinetics in this diffuse lobular cancer is predominately progressive in the 3:00 axis, at the site of the palpable mass.

- Plate 9.4I—However, the kinetics are much more heterogeneous in the inner upper quadrant, where they are demonstrates predominantly plateau type, but with small regions of washout.

DISCUSSION

On sonography, many invasive lobular carcinomas can present as discrete hypoechoic shadowing lesions; however, as in this case, some can have more non specific findings. Mammographically, invasive lobular carcinomas are notorious for failing detection because of the subtle nature of findings. They can be subtle on MRI as well, but are, in general, much more easily seen on MRI than on digital mammography. Learning to recognize the subtle signs is important. Look for asymmetry with the other breast. The delayed scans may be more revealing as to the true nature and size of these lesions, as many lobular carcinomas enhance progressively.

• Plate 5

HISTORY

A 67-year-old woman presents with abnormal MRI obtained for high-risk screening for positive family history which demonstrated an faintly enhancing nodule in the left lower outer quadrant. Digital mammography and sonography were initially negative. Targeted (second-look) US, however, demonstrated the presence of a hypoechoic shadowing area thought to correspond to the abnormality on MRI and US-guided biopsy was performed. This demonstrated an invasive lobular carcinoma. She subsequently underwent lumpectomy with sentinel node biopsy, which demonstrated a 1.2-cm invasive lobular carcinoma and negative sentinel lymph nodes.

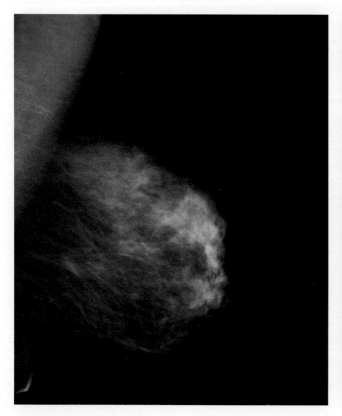

Plate 9.5A

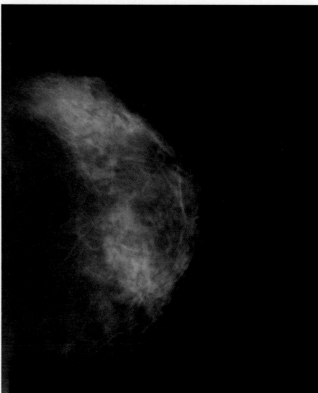

Plate 9.5B

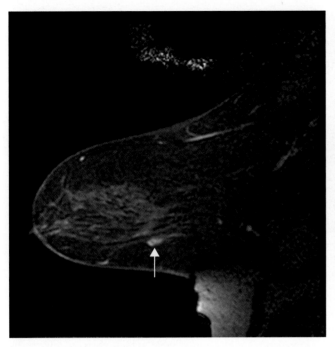

Plate 9.5C

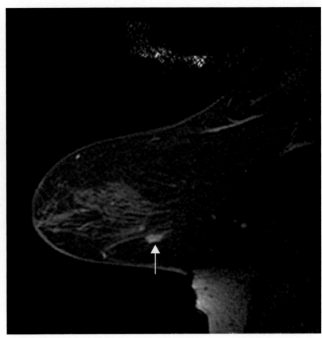

Plate 9.5D

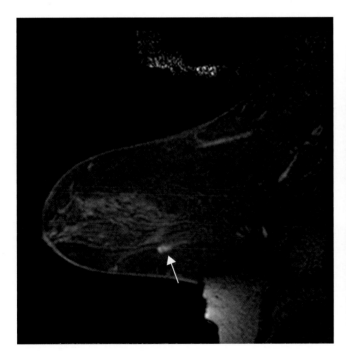

Plate 9.5E

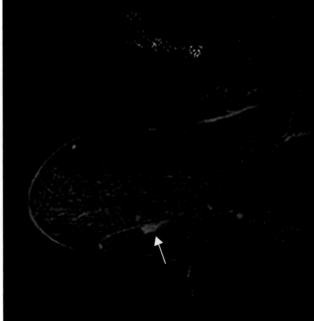

Plate 9.5F

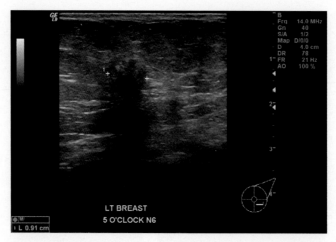

Plate 9.5G

FINDINGS

- Plates 9.5A–B—Digital mammographic images of the left breast interpreted as dense breasts with no suspicious findings. In retrospect, there is a patch of soft-tissue density seen in the lower breast in the mediolateral oblique view, which corresponds to the abnormality subsequently seen on high-risk screening MRI.

- Plates 9.5C–F—MRI demonstrating an irregular enhancing nodule in the lower breast, seen best on the fourth series subtracted image (F).

- Plate 9.5G—Demonstrates targeted second-look US with poorly defined hypoechoic shadowing region corresponding to the MRI abnormality.

DISCUSSION

Again, findings that are obvious on MRI can be easily overlooked or undetectable on digital mammography and sonography. It is a well-established fact that approximately 15% of carcinomas are missed on screening digital mammography, and an even higher percentage are obscured in dense breasts. MRI screening is now being performed for high-risk women, and we are discovering many of these previously overlooked lesions. We have also noted, not unexpectedly, that a fair number of these lesions are also being detected on "clinical or mammographic problem solving" MRI exams in average-risk dense breasted women.

• Plate 1

HISTORY

A 57-year-old woman who was undergoing magnetic resonance imaging (MRI) screening for positive family history as well as personal history of right breast carcinoma, who had been treated with breast conservation therapy 5 years prior. Her mammogram was negative with the exception of postlumpectomy changes. Her ultrasound (US) was noncontributory. The MRI demonstrated retroareolar linear enhancement as well new small adjacent grouped enhancing foci. In a postlumpectomy patient, those findings are especially suspicious and warrant biopsy. A core biopsy was performed and demonstrated atypical ductal hyperplasia. An excisional biopsy was performed and demonstrated a 1.8-cm area of ductal carcinoma in situ (DCIS). Due to a previous breast conservation surgery and radiation therapy, mastectomy was performed. Final pathology demonstrated multiple foci of DCIS within a lactiferous duct.

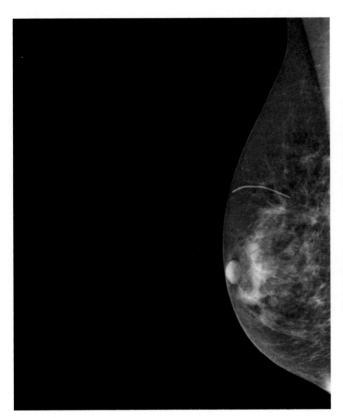

Plate 10.1A

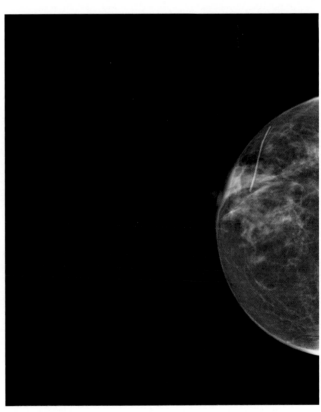

Plate 10.1B

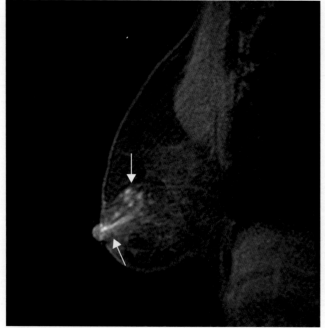

Plate 10.1C

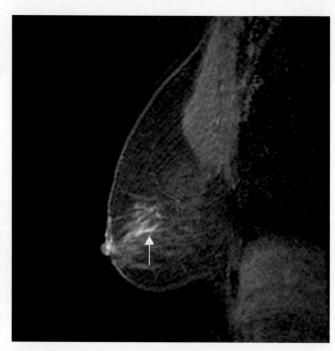

Plate 10.1D

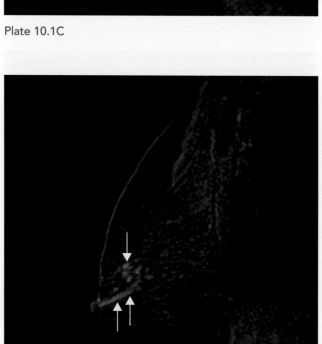

Plate 10.1E

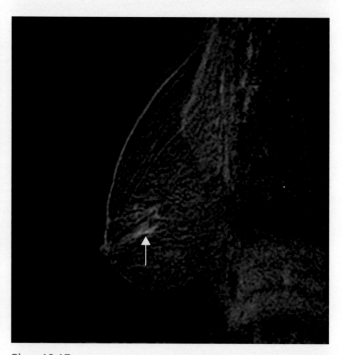

Plate 10.1F

FINDINGS

- Plates 10.1A–B—Demonstrates right mammogram with a scar marker at lumpectomy site.
- Plates 10.1C–F—Postcontrast and subtracted sagital images, which show linear, retroareolar enhancement and clustered enhancing foci. The linear enhancement travels from central aspect of breast to the nipple. At the posterior aspect of the linear enhancement, there is some branching noted, suggesting a ductal configuration, which is highly suspicious for DCIS/recurrence (arrows D, F).

DISCUSSION

Although history of breast carcinoma in and of itself does not meet the American Cancer Society's guidelines for high risk status, digital mammography, sonography, and clinical exam of postlumpectomy/post-radiation patients is fraught with difficulty. In order to find a recurrence before invasion or lymph node metastasis occurs, MRI screening can be considered in select patients, especially when mammogram/US/clinical exam is limited. The presence of linear enhancement that extends to the nipple in a postlumpectomy breast is extremely suspicious. It may, however, be difficult to biopsy; due to perpendicular orientation of the lesion with respect to the needle, only a small sample of actual tumor is often retrieved. If the result is benign and no retroareolar ductal ectasia is seen on STIR or precontrast scans, the pathology may be discordant. One can try to angle the needle anteriorly and posteriorly to get as much tissue as possible. Duct ectasia (dilated ducts containing fluid or hemorrhagic/proteinaceous debris) with periductal inflammation may demonstrate periductal linear enhancement that mimics this appearance of DCIS. Always check your STIR/T2 and precontrast series to see if this is a potential benign explanation for this appearance before you recommend biopsy.

• Plate 2

HISTORY

A 42-year-old woman who was undergoing annual high-risk screening breast MRI for personal and family history of premenopausal breast cancer. She has had a right breast lumpectomy and radiation therapy. Annual digital mammography and sonography were negative. On screening MRI, new small enhancing nodule was noted anterior to the right breast lumpectomy site. MRI-guided core biopsy demonstrated DCIS and atypia. She underwent a right mastectomy and TRAM reconstruction and a left reduction mammoplasty to match. Final pathology demonstrates a small area of DCIS and negative nodes. She continued annual MRI screening of the left. Two years later, she demonstrated an area of branching linear enhancement in the left breast, which was also found to represent DCIS on MRI core biopsy. She opted for a second mastectomy.

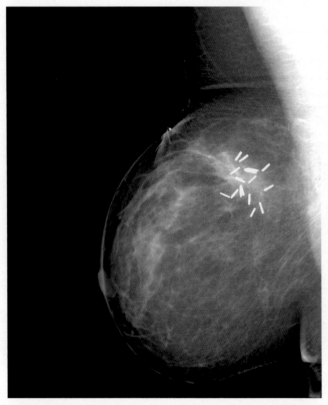

Plate 10.2A

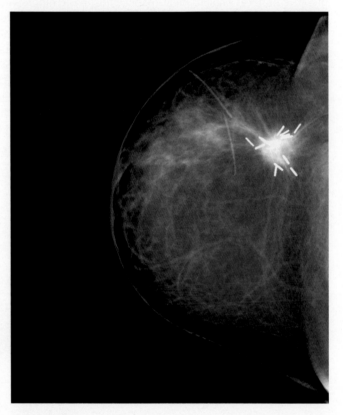

Plate 10.2B

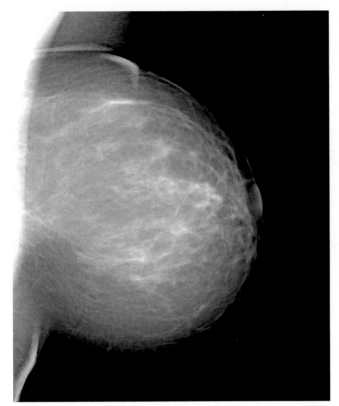

Plate 10.2C

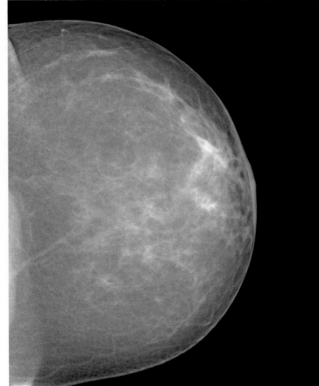

Plate 10.2D

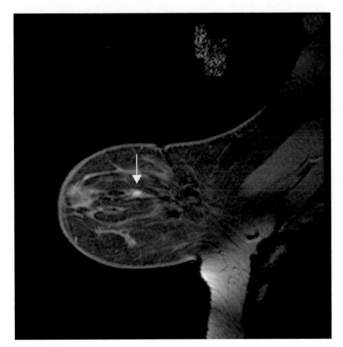

Plate 10.2E

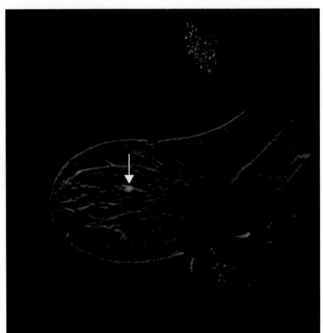

Plate 10.2F

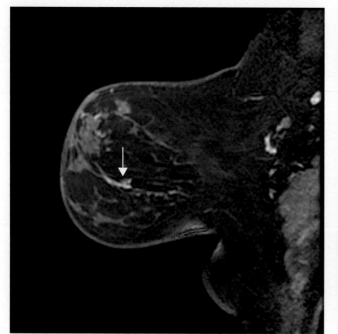

Plate 10.2G

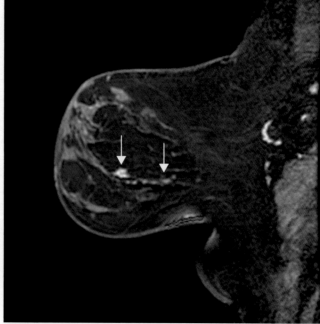

Plate 10.2H

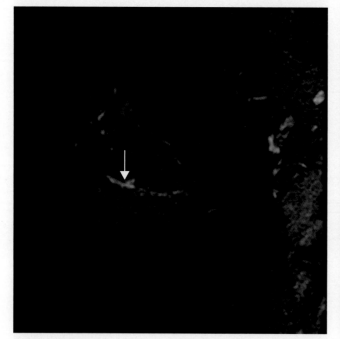

Plate 10.2I

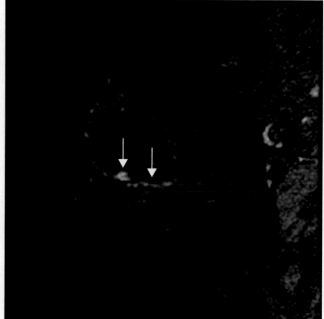

Plate 10.2J

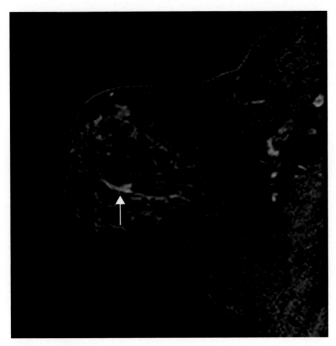

Plate 10.2K

FINDINGS

- Plates 10.2A–B—Postlumpectomy/radiation with numerous clips at the lumpectomy site (right digital mammography).

- Plates 10.2C–D—Normal large left breast digital mammography demonstrating predominantly fatty tissue (pre-reduction).

- Plates 10.2E–F—Right MRI; 4-mm new enhancing right breast nodule anterior to lumpectomy site.

- Plates 10.2G–K—Left MRI. Demonstrates the long area of linear branching enhancement with several foci lining up in a ductal distribution. The enhancing foci seen on 1st postcontrast early images coalesce into a more continuous line of enhancement on later (4th postcontrast) images.

DISCUSSION

This unfortunate young woman initially presented with a palpable right lump in her late 30s. Even though her breasts are fatty, she did benefit from MRI, as it detected a small right recurrence and new left primary lesion in the early noninvasive stage (stage 0). A normal postradiation breast should have very little if any enhancement. Any new enhancement should be viewed with suspicion. If not consistent with fat necrosis (and demonstrating fat within the lesion on nonfat-suppressed series), any new MRI lesion in a postlumpectomy breast should be biopsied. Residual, stable, or decreasing enhancement at the lumpectomy site may be seen, but this should be faint, thin, and circumferential, and without evidence of mass.

• Plate 3

HISTORY

A 72-year-old woman who presents with her first screening breast MRI for personal (4 years prior) history as well as family history of breast cancer. She was treated with breast conservation and radiation therapy. Her MRI demonstrated a suspicious faintly enhancing area medial to the right breast lumpectomy site and an area of irregular linear enhancement on the left. Breast MRI core biopsies demonstrated a right invasive ductal carcinoma and DCIS on the left. She underwent bilateral mastectomies. Final pathology was a 1.5-cm invasive ductal on right and 0.5-cm DCIS on the left with negative bilateral sentinel lymph nodes.

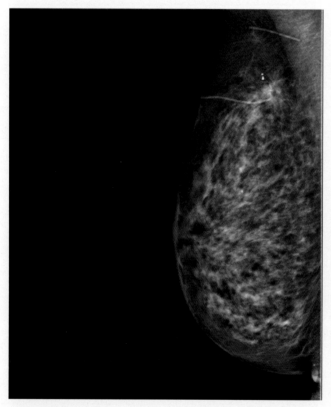

Plate 10.3A

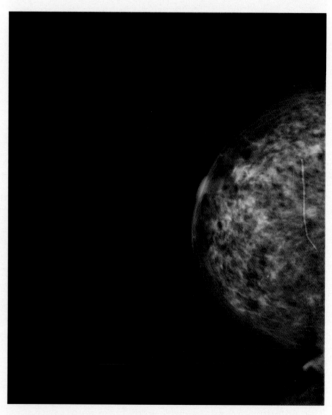

Plate 10.3B

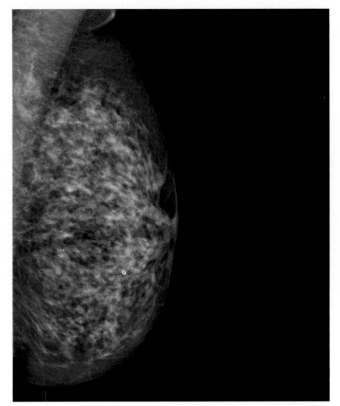

Plate 10.3C

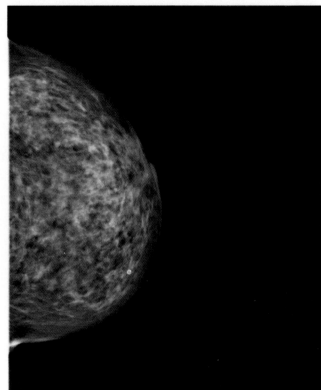

Plate 10.3D

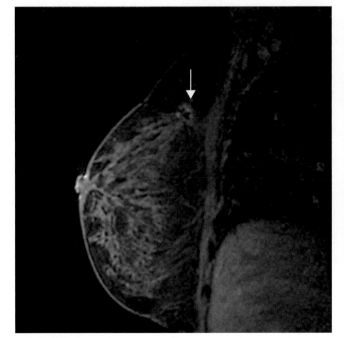

Plate 10.3E

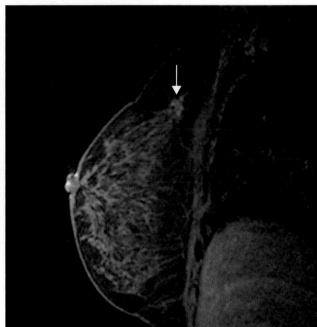

Plate 10.3F

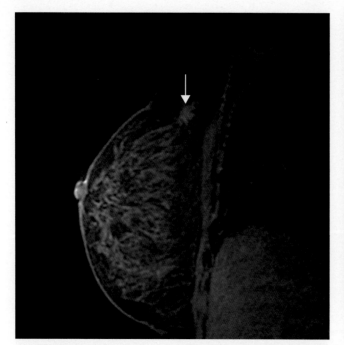

Plate 10.3G

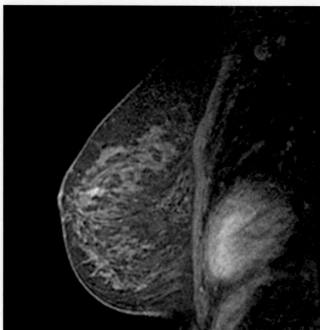

Plate 10.3H

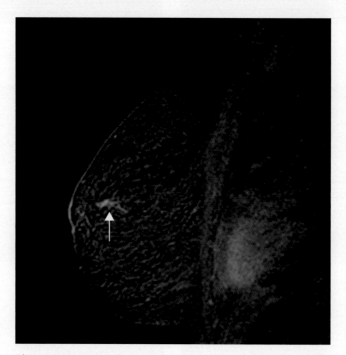

Plate 10.3I

FINDINGS

- Plates 10.3A–D—Bilateral mammogram demonstrating heterogeneously dense parenchyma as well as postlumpectomy changes in the right upper breast with stable coarse/dystrophic calcifications.

- Plate 10.3E—Lumpectomy site with minimal faint rim enhancement.

- Plates 10.3F–G—Irregular nodular mass-like area of enhancement adjacent and medial to the lumpectomy site suspicious for recurrence.

- Plates 10.3H–I—Also noted (in the opposite breast) is an irregular area of linear enhancement, best seen on subtracted images (I).

DISCUSSION

Findings on MRI may lead to complicated workups. Bilateral MRI core biopsies are difficult to perform, as scanning through both breasts can result in contrast dissipating before accurate targeting has been performed. It is usually better to perform bilateral biopsy on separate days, unless a clinical situation or patient inconvenience requires a same-day procedure. Although the most concerning lesion was in the right breast, other suspicious findings should not be overlooked. We will usually biopsy the most suspicious lesion first, and based on that pathology, decide if less suspicious lesions also need sampling. In general, if the most suspicious area in a patient's breast is adequately and accurately biopsied and proves to be benign, then any remaining less suspicious appearing areas are also more likely benign, and can be safely followed with short-term follow-up exams, as BIRADS 3 (probably benign) lesions. Any change on follow-up exams, of course, should prompt immediate intervention/biopsy.

• Plate 4

HISTORY

A 50-year-old woman with history of left breast lumpectomy, 9 years prior undergoing high-risk screening with MRI. Screening digital mammography demonstrated new suspicious clustered calcifications, and screening MRI demonstrates corresponding tiny, brightly enhancing foci in a linear distribution. The post-MRI demonstrates the cavity of the stereo biopsy is in the same region of the MRI abnormality. Pathology demonstrated DCIS and patient underwent mastectomy. Final pathology demonstrated a 5-mm invasive ductal carcinoma and negative sentinel nodes.

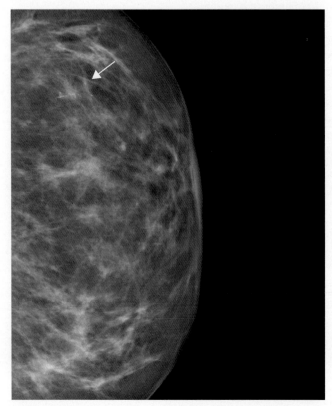

Plate 10.4A

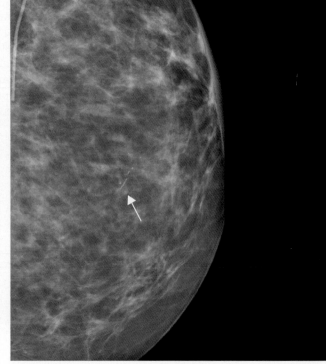

Plate 10.4B

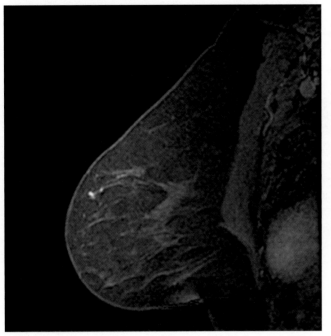

Plate 10.4C

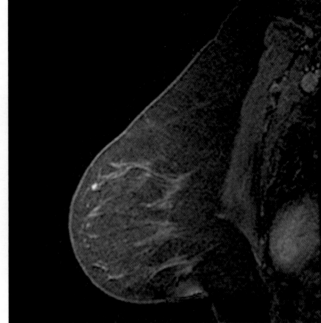

Plate 10.4D

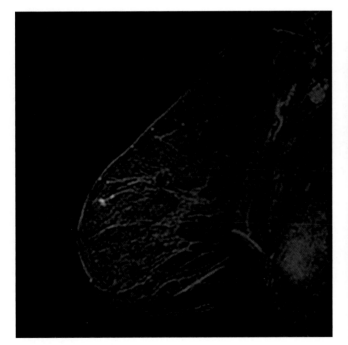

Plate 10.4E

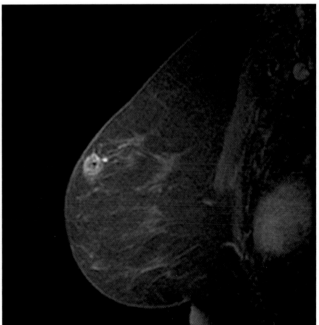

Plate 10.4F

FINDINGS

- Plates 10.4A–B—Digital mammography demonstrated linear casting type calcifications suspicious for DCIS in a postlumpectomy breast.
- Plates 10.4C–E—MRI demonstrating corresponding tiny intensely enhancing foci, in a linear distribution.
- Plate 10.4F—Stereo cavity with one enhancing focus remaining, posterior to the biopsy cavity.

DISCUSSION

Although in the average patient tiny enhancing foci can be benign, in a postradiation breast, these foci are suspicious, even if small, and especially if new and intensely, rapidly enhancing. Other than in benign intramammary nodes, rapid intense enhancement is a suspicious finding. Since postradiation breasts are usually devoid of background glandular enhancement, even a small recurrence may be quite obvious.

• **Plate 5**

HISTORY

A 69-year-old woman with a history of left upper outer quadrant breast carcinoma treated with lumpectomy and radiation therapy, who underwent MRI for questionable mammographic findings in the contra lateral (right) breast. Incidentally noted in the postlumpectomy left breast are two adjacent tiny enhancing in the 12:00 axis. These findings were interpreted as BIRADS (probably benign), and 6-month follow-up MRI was recommended. An MRI core biopsy 6 months later demonstrated invasive ductal carcinoma. Subsequent mastectomy demonstrated an 6-mm ductal carcinoma with negative lymph nodes.

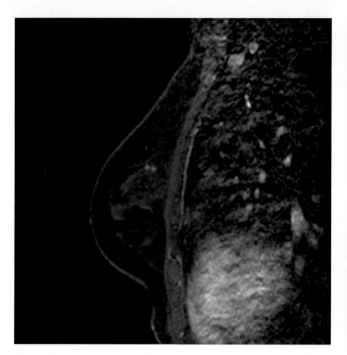

Plate 10.5A

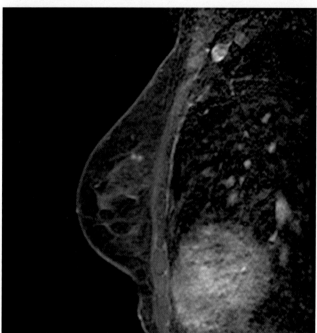

Plate 10.5B

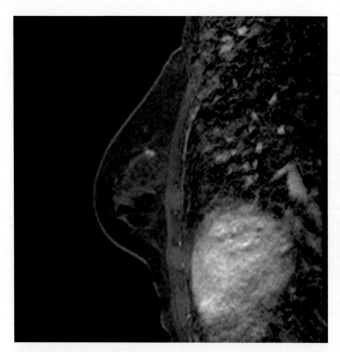

Plate 10.5C

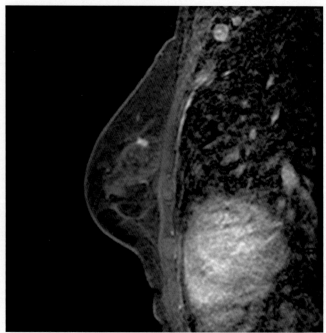

Plate 10.5D

FINDINGS

- Plates 10.5A–B—Baseline sagittal postcontrast first and fourth series demonstrate two intensely enhancing foci, several centimeters away from the lumpectomy site. Enhancing foci are unusual in a postradiation breast. Notice the slight "bleeding" of the margins and "blossoming"/enlargement of these two foci on the fourth series (B), which should increase your level of suspicion.

- Plates 10.5C–D—Six months later, each of the foci have enlarged slightly and are nearly coalescent on the first postcontrast series (C). On the last postcontrast series (D), the true nature of this lesion is evident, as the two foci appear coalesced into a mass and a spiculated margin is now clearly visible.

DISCUSSION

Postradiation breasts typically demonstrate no enhancement, so even a tiny focus of enhancement can be significant, especially if it is intense. As discussed previously, we have found "blossoming" of the margin to be more suggestive of a malignant lesion than a benign well-encapsulated one.

Six-month follow-up for MRI can be warranted in some circumstances; anecdotally, we have found malignancy to appear to change more rapidly and declare its true nature on 6 month follow-up MRI than on 6-month follow-up digital mammography or sonography.

Standard accepted normal, postsurgical enhancement at a benign biopsy site should last for only 6 months; at a lumpectomy site after radiation, this extends to 18 months. However, spiculated or mass-like enhancement or increasing area of enhancement should be viewed with suspicion, even within the first 18 months postradiation.

In contrast, although standard teaching is post-lumpectomy enhancement should resolve in 18 months, those with seromas can demonstrate thin faint rim enhancement for years. As long as the enhancement is minimal, stable, or diminishing, follow-up is likely a reasonable option, as we have yet to have a positive biopsy in these cases. Also, this type of post-lumpectomy residual enhancement usually displays progressive kinetics, not wash-out.

• Plate 6

HISTORY

A 74-year-old with history of left breast carcinoma treated with lumpectomy and radiation therapy 21 years ago. She developed a new nodule (arrows) seen on one view only in the postlumpectomy breast on mammogram. Her mammogram was limited by marked post-surgical deformity, and this area was too posterior to allow for stereotactic biopsy. MRI was performed for problem solving, and demonstrated an 8-mm ring-enhancing nodule in the posterior central breast, posterior to lumpectomy site. It did not contain fat on the nonfat-suppressed series, and did not contain fluid on the STIR series, nor did it contain hemorrhagic or proteinaceous debris on precontrast series. (These findings would have suggested a benign etiology). MRI core biopsy was therefore performed and demonstrated an atypical papillary lesion. Subsequent excision yielded an intracystic carcinoma, and the patient underwent mastectomy.

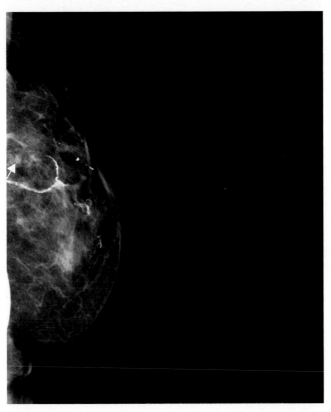

Plate 10.6A

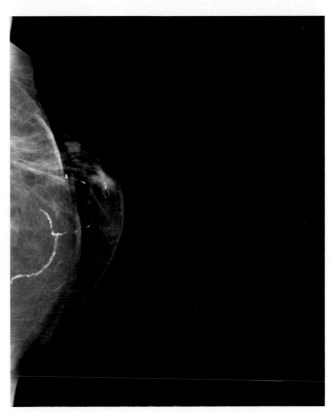

Plate 10.6B

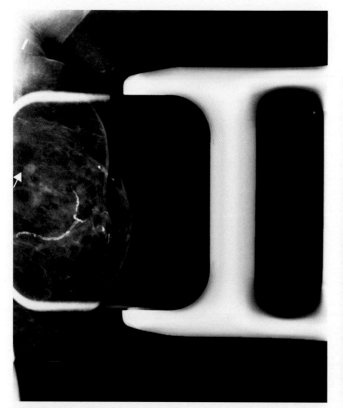

Plate 10.6C

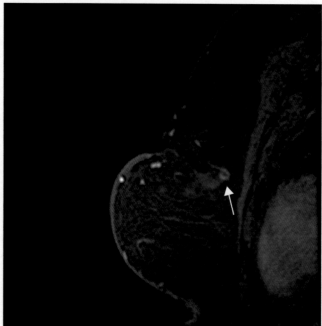

Plate 10.6D

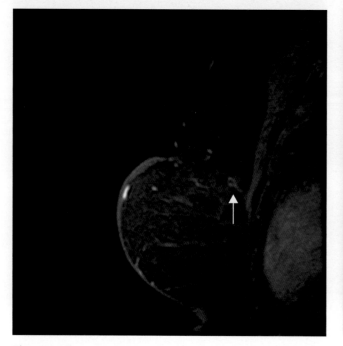

Plate 10.6E

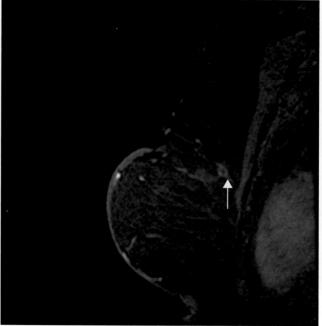

Plate 10.6F

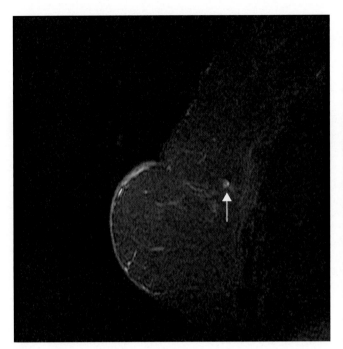

Plate 10.6G

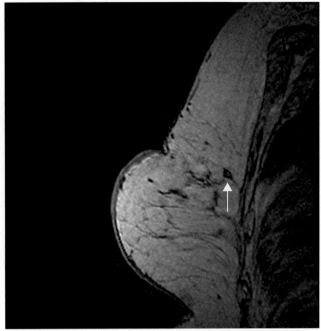

Plate 10.6H

FINDINGS

- Plates 10.6A–C—Digital mammography images. A new small non-specific nodular density is seen.
- Plates 10.6D–F—Postcontrast series. Ring enhancement is seen.
- Plate 10.6G—STIR image. Only a small amount of fluid intensity is present in the posterior aspect of this nodule.
- Plate 10.6H—Nonfat-suppressed image. The nodule is not fat-filled.

DISCUSSION

Intracystic carcinomas can be difficult to distinguish from cysts. Differentiating features include irregular or thick rim, spiculation or adjacent linear enhancement.

Ring- or rim-enhancing lesions near a surgical site frequently represent fat necrosis. Use the additional series other than the postcontrast (i.e., precontrast, STIR/T2, nonfat-suppressed series) to exclude benign etiologies. If there is no definitive benign explanation for a new mammographic finding, biopsy must be performed. In this case, location and post-surgical deformity made stereotactic biopsy as well as mammographic needle localization difficult. Without knowing the location of the lesion via MRI guided clip placement, localization would have been difficult or impossible, as it was a one view–only finding. Rim-enhancing lesions containing fat are consistent with fat necrosis. Rim-enhancing lesions containing fluid (on T2/STIR series) are consistent with cysts. Rim-enhancing lesions containing hemorrhagic or proteinaceous material (bright on precontrast T1-weighted images) are consistent with hemorrhagic or proteinaceous debris-filled cysts.

• Plate 7

HISTORY

A 45-year-old woman who had right breast carcinoma treated with bilateral mastectomy and reconstruction 5 years prior. She developed a palpable abnormality in the left breast with no corresponding mammographic or sonographic finding. MRI was performed for clinical problem solving; a vitamin E capsule was placed over the palpable area of concern. No MRI finding was noted to explain the left palpable finding, which is now attributed to a fold in the prosthesis. However, in the right axillary tail, there are, irregular, lobulated enhancing mass(es) with adjacent enlarged lymph nodes. Targeted US demonstrated two adjacent hypoechoic irregular shadowing areas. US-guided core biopsy demonstrated invasive ductal carcinoma.

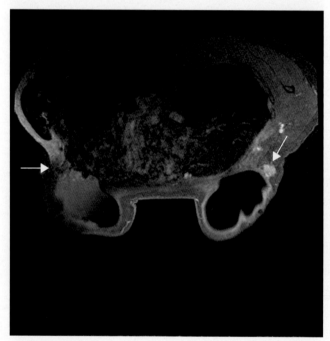

Plate 10.7A

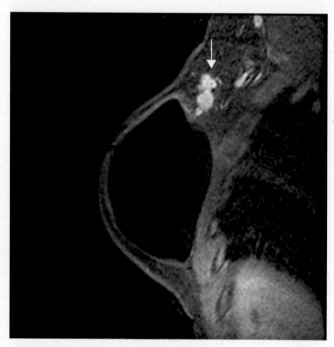

Plate 10.7B

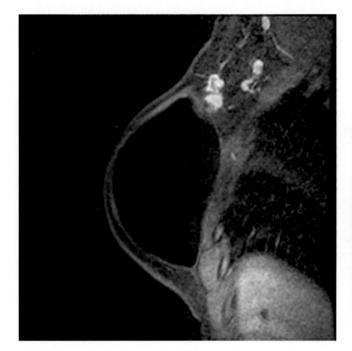

Plate 10.7C

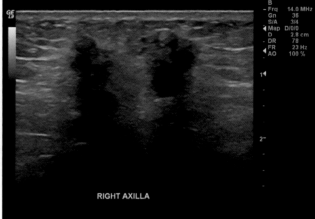

Plate 10.7D

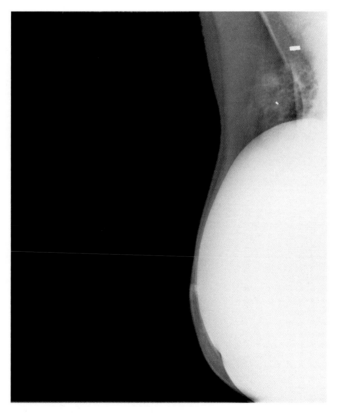

Plate 10.7E

FINDINGS

- Plates 10.7A–C—Axial and sagittal postcontrast images demonstrating the vitamin E capsule in the left axillary tail and the dumbbell-shaped mass in the right axillary tail.
- Plate 10.7D—US image demonstrating irregular hypoechoic suspicious masses in the right axillary region of the reconstructed breast.
- Plate 10.7E—Angulated mammographic image showing implant and postbiopsy clip in the right axillary tail. A larger surgical clip is also noted more superiorly, from prior node dissection.

DISCUSSION

Gene positive patients postbilateral mastectomies have a 90% (not a 100%) decreased risk of developing breast cancer. The presence of prostheses severely limits clinical evaluation for occurrence of disease and will almost always obscure the detection of disease on mammogram. Women who are gene positive and have had mastectomy should be considered for MRI screening, especially if they have had reconstructive surgery. Although MRI screening in this setting is still being studied as to its efficacy, it may become a standard recommendation in the future.

• Plate 1

HISTORY

A 66-year-old woman with history of complicated digital mammography and sonography, and multiple previous benign biopsies, now with a questionable mass versus asymmetric density in the *right* breast. Magnetic resonance imaging (MRI) was performed for mammographic problem solving.

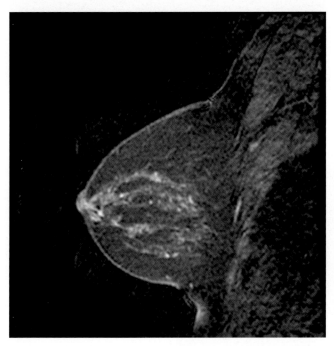

Plate 11.1A

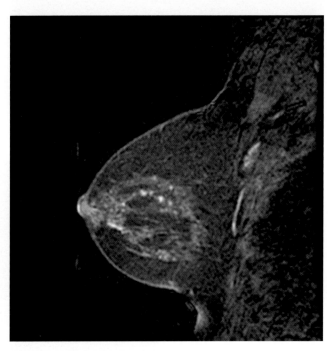

Plate 11.1B

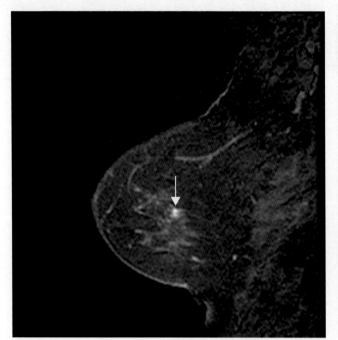

Plate 11.1C

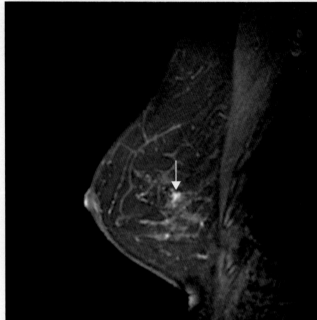

Plate 11.1D

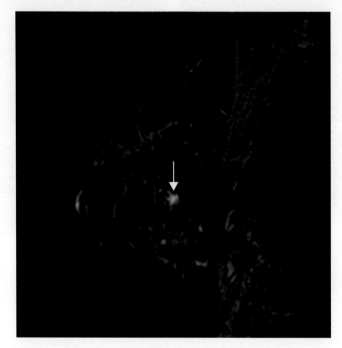

Plate 11.1E

FINDINGS

- Plates 11.1A–C—Both breasts demonstrate numerous enhancing foci, the largest which was seen in the contralateral (*left*) outer breast (4 mm, see arrow image C) for which 6-month follow-up MRI was recommended.

- Plates 11.D–E—Postcontrast and subtraction images at 6-month follow-up the left outer focus has enlarged slightly and now demonstrates small radiating spicules and an irregular margin. MRI core biopsy was recommended, and pathology demonstrated invasive ductal carcinoma. She underwent lumpectomy and sentinel node biopsy. Final pathology—a 4-mm invasive mucinous ductal carcinoma with negative sentinel nodes.

DISCUSSION

Usually when interpreting breast MRI, we focus attention only on enhancing lesions measuring 5 mm or greater. While this is usually appropriate, because the vast majority of tiny enhancing foci are benign (glandular), these lesions cannot always be dismissed so easily. If all the foci in both breast are small, but one stands out in size (larger), a short-term follow-up exam or biopsy may be warranted. Another feature that may raise suspicion is washout kinetics, or a pattern of kinetics differing from the foci in the rest of the breast. In patients with high-risk status, a more aggressive recommendation may be required. This lesion was not biopsied initially, as the patient had already undergone many benign biopsies and had no other risk factors. Furthermore, the questioned abnormality on digital mammography was in the contralateral breast, so this focus represented an incidental finding. The rapid change in the lesion in the 6-month interval, however, made the diagnosis much more obvious.

• Plate 2

HISTORY

A 58-year-old with history of contralateral (left) breast carcinoma treated with mastectomy and numerous negative US-guided core biopsies on the right breast. She was undergoing annual high-risk screening MRI for personal and family history of breast carcinoma.

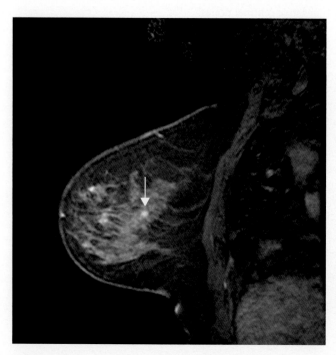

Plate 11.2A

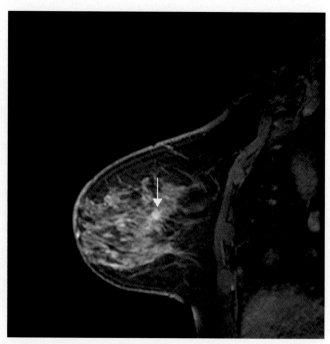

Plate 11.2B

FINDINGS

* Plate 11.2A—Demonstrated a new 3-mm enhancing focus, on a background of numerous scattered enhancing foci. Due to her history, short-term MRI follow-up was recommended.
* Plate 11.2B—At the 6-month follow-up, the focus has increased in size as well as developed superior spiculations. Core needle biopsy demonstrated an invasive ductal carcinoma. Lumpectomy demonstrated a 6-mm invasive carcinoma with adjacent ductal carcinoma in situ (DCIS).

DISCUSSION

Although this focus was not significantly larger than the other foci in this breast, the change from the prior exams along with her high-risk status prompted closer surveillance. The rapid change in appearance (within 6 months) markedly raises the level of suspicion.

• Plate 3

HISTORY

A 43-year-old with high-risk MRI screening for family history of breast cancer who presented with a small enhancing nodule or focus in the right upper outer quadrant. A targeted ultrasound and subsequent US-guided core biopsy were performed. These demonstrated the presence of a fibroadenoma. A 6-month follow-up was performed as a postbiopsy check. The nodule appeared slightly large more intensely enhancing, and with spiculations and some nearby new (inferior) grouped enhancing foci. The biopsy clip was approximately 1 cm from the nodule. Rebiopsy was performed with MRI guidance. Core biopsy results demonstrated invasive ductal carcinoma. She underwent lumpectomy with sentinel node biopsy. Final pathology showed an invasive ductal carcinoma as well as an adjacent small fibroadenoma.

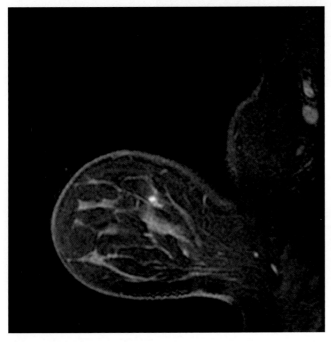

Plate 11.3A

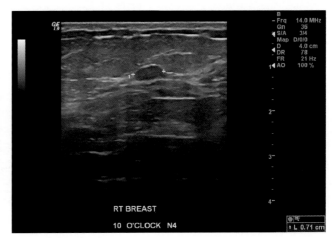

Plate 11.3B

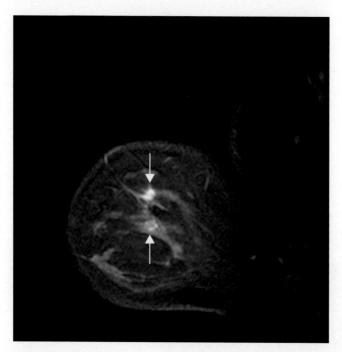

Plate 11.3C

FINDINGS

- Plate 11.3A—Baseline screening MRI. Showing small ovoid enhancing right upper outer guided nodule.
- Plate 11.3B—US lesion—smooth ovoid hypo echoic nodule corresponding is size, shape and location to the enhancing structure on MRI.
- Plate 11.3C—Six-month follow-up MRI, demonstrate enlargement of the nodule, spiculation of the lateral edge of the nodule, and new enhancing foci inferior to the nodule.

DISCUSSION

We routinely recommend 6-month follow-up imaging after core needle biopsy. This is especially important to perform in the setting of targeted US biopsies. Despite careful correlation of size, shape, axis of lesion, quadrant and distance from nipple, an abnormality identified on US may *not* represent the same lesion seen on MRI. If feasible, after the initial US core biopsy for an MRI lesion, a repeat MRI can be used to check clip placement. In addition, for lesions <1 to 1.5 cm, we prefer to perform MRI core biopsies rather than targeted US-guided needle biopsies, in order to avoid this type of situation.

• Plate 4

HISTORY

A 47-year-old with high-risk screening MRI. On baseline MRI, a small enhancing focus was thought to possibly represent a benign intramammary lymph node, and a 6-month follow-up was recommended (Birads 3). In retrospect, on the fourth postcontrast series, the margins were slightly less distinct compared to the first series and the focus had "blossomed" slightly in size. At 6-month follow-up, the lesion increased in size and demonstrated central clearing (ring enhancement) seen most prominently on the fourth series, which raised the level of suspicion. MRI-guided needle biopsy was recommended. Final pathology demonstrated a 5-mm invasive ductal carcinoma.

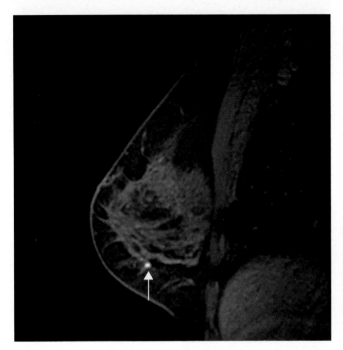

Plate 11.4A

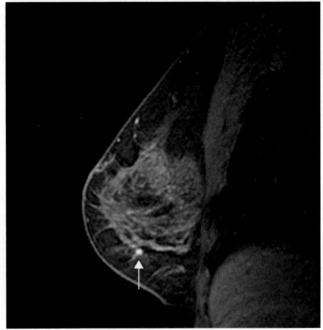

Plate 11.4B

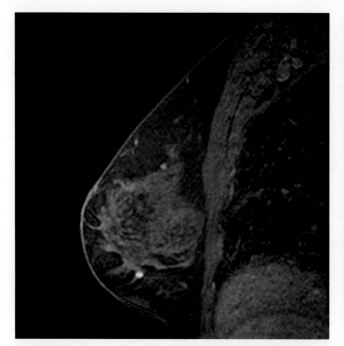

Plate 11.4C

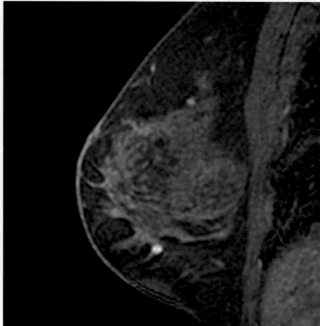

Plate 11.4D

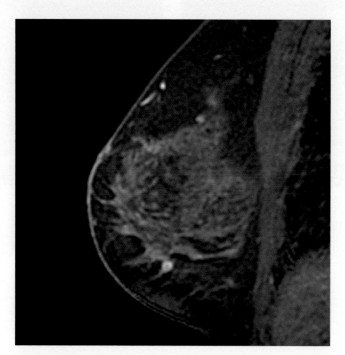

Plate 11.4E

FINDINGS

- Plate 11.4A—First postcontrast series from the initial exam.
- Plate 11.4B—Last postcontrast series from the initial exam.
- Plates 11.4C–D—Six months later, first postcontrast series.
- Plate 11.4E—Six months later, last postcontrast series.

DISCUSSION

Again, any lesion that is of concern but not suspicious enough to warrant biopsy may reveal its true nature within a 6-month follow-up. We have found a greater incidence of positive CAs on 6-month follow-up MRI than on 6-month follow-up mammograms or ultrasounds. Traditional teaching and guidelines states that BIRADS 3 digital mammography recommendation should be applied to cases where the risk of a lesion being breast cancer is <1% to 2%. The incidence of breast cancer at 6-month follow-up MRI varies greatly according to the current literature but is likely somewhat higher than the <1% to 2% rule used in digital mammography. The role of "BIRADS 3—probably benign, recommend 6-month follow-up" in MRI interpretation is still being developed. This situation is complicated by the difficulty in obtaining precertification for 6-month follow-up MRIs, as insurance companies have not uniformly recognized the BIRADS nomenclature/reporting for MRI exams.

These plates either had no magnetic resonance imaging (MRI) findings or subtle MRI findings only visible in retrospect, but patients did ultimately have a positive diagnosis. Therefore, these cases are included as instructive, in that one must consider all imaging features to determine further intervention, and should not rely only on the MRI findings.

• Plate 1

HISTORY

A 60-year-old woman who presents with a weakly positive family history for breast cancer. She is on hormone replacement therapy. She has recent abnormal sonogram with numerous cysts and small hypoechoic probably benign nodules, as well as a suspicious hypoechoic shadowing lesion measuring 7 mm. MRI was recommended for further evaluation, and the ultrasound was officially interpreted as BIRADS "0" incomplete exam. The prior ultrasound (US) study was not available to the radiologist who interpreted the MRI. Her MRI was interpreted as BIRADS 3 (probably benign) for numerous small enhancing foci/nodules. When the patient returned, approximately 6 months later for follow-up, all studies were repeated, and despite no change in MRI findings, the proper follow-up recommendation for the suspicious US finding was made. US-guided core biopsy of the shadowing lesion demonstrated a 7-mm invasive lobular carcinoma.

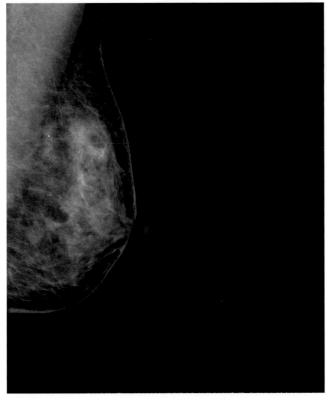

Plate 12.1A

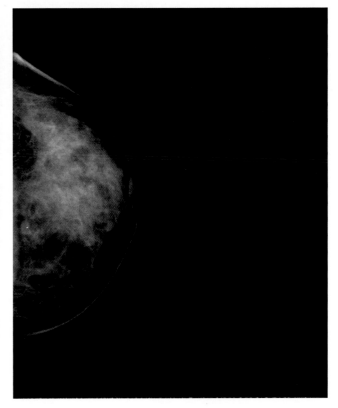

Plate 12.1B

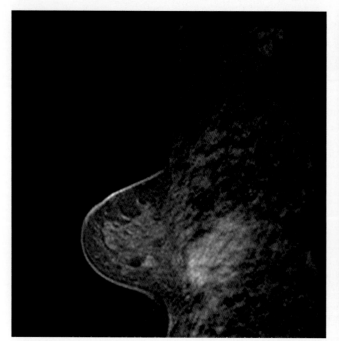

Plate 12.1C

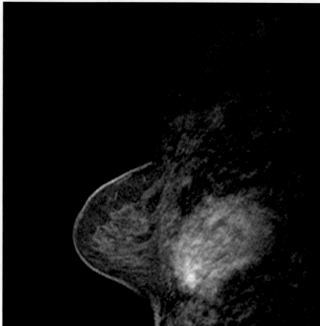

Plate 12.1D

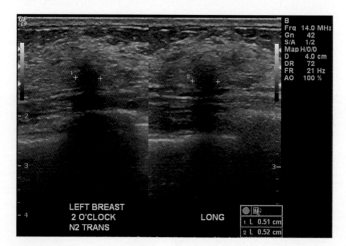

Plate 12.1E

FINDINGS

- Plates 12.1A–B—Digital mammography demonstrating dense breasts; no mammographic evidence of malignancy.
- Plates 12.1C–D—No enhancement in left upper outer breast to correspond to US finding on early or delayed images.
- Plate 12.1E—US demonstrating a 7-mm hypoechoic shadowing lesion.

DISCUSSION

When reviewing MRI after digital mammography/sonography, the results and recommendations of all prior imaging should be addressed in the MRI reading. Be sure to look at all previous images and comment on the recommendation, not just for the MRI but for the images prior (including mammogram and US) that may have lead to the MRI being requested. The MRI interpretation is viewed as the final reading and opinion on the entire case. Clinicians and patients cannot be expected to understand the implication of "hypoechoic shadowing nodule" or other nomenclature used by radiologists to indicate that a biopsy is warranted. If outside images are not available to review, insist on being provided with the outside radiology report. A negative MRI does not rule out the possibility of a malignancy that can be seen mammographically or sonographically. Although MRI is the most sensitive modality, a suspicious lesion seen in any modality should be evaluated with biopsy, as the absence of MRI findings does not entirely exclude the presence of malignancy.

Although MRI is the most sensitive exam for detection of breast cancer, it can fail to detect a very small percentage of cases, including some invasive lobulars can as visible on ultrasound, some cases of DCIS seen as calcifications on digital mammography, and some small palpable carcinomas.

• Plate 2

HISTORY

A 63-year-old presented with an abnormal screening mammogram (no risk factors). She had a small new cluster of calcifications in the right breast, and a nonspecific nodularity in the left breast with no corresponding abnormality on US. MRI was recommended to evaluate left breast nodularity. The mammogram was interpreted as BIRADS 0. MRI demonstrated a benign-appearing intramammary lymph node in the left breast, and no findings in the right breast.

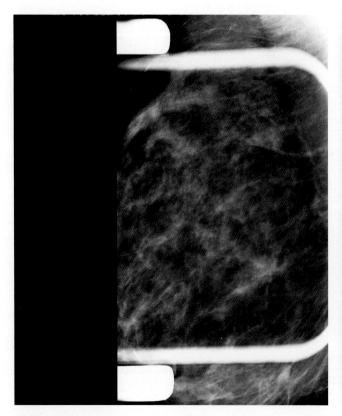

Plate 12.2A

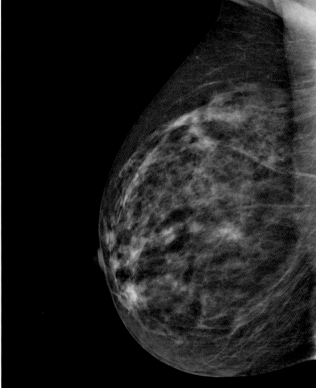

Plate 12.2B

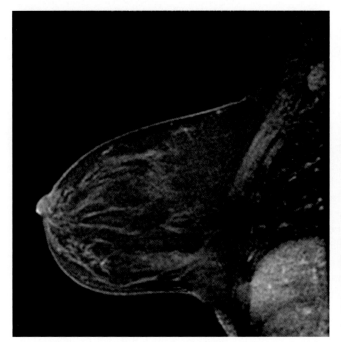

Plate 12.2C

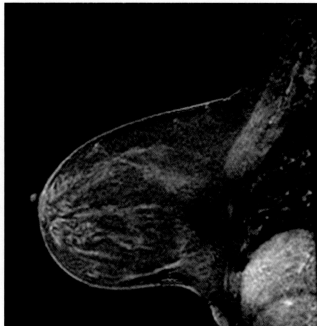

Plate 12.2D

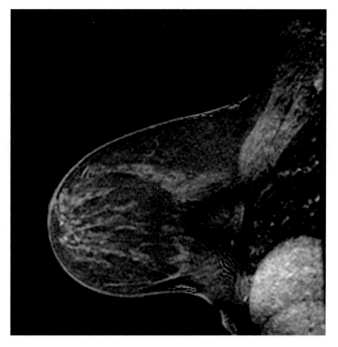

Plate 12.2E

FINDINGS

- Plates 12.2A–B—Mammogram demonstrating a small cluster of heterogeneous calcifications that were new compared to prior year.
- Plates 12.2C–E—MRI with no suspicious corresponding areas of enhancement in the right breast.

DISCUSSION

The American College of Radiology recommends *against* using a BIRADs "0" impression when interpreting a diagnostic mammogram and requesting MRI, and this case is a good example of why not to do this! Because biopsy was not specifically recommended for the new tiny cluster of right breast calcifications, and the outside report was not reviewed by the radiologist interpreting the MRI, the essentially negative MRI report was assumed by the referring clinician to be the final word on the case. Fortunately, when the patient returned for a 6-month follow-up exam, this situation became apparent and stereotactic biopsy of right breast calcifications was performed. This demonstrated ductal carcinoma in situ (DCIS) and subsequent lumpectomy yielded only a few millimeters of residual DCIS.

If you are interpreting an MRI that has been recommended for mammographic and/or sonographic abnormalities, it is imperative that you review these images (or at least the reports) and address these findings in your impression. If the other studies have been incorrectly labeled as BIRADS 0, you should reassign correct BIRADS to these exams whenever possible. A negative MRI is not uncommon when a small focus of DCIS or small invasive lobular carcinoma are present. In these settings, you must recommend a biopsy despite the absence of suspicious MRI findings.

• Plate 3

HISTORY

A 75-year-old with a new nipple retraction and periareolar skin thickening seen clinically and on digital mammography. Her initial US was negative. An MRI was performed and demonstrated faint stippled segmental retroareolar enhancement. The differential diagnosis included glandular enhancement, but in the setting of suspicious mammographic and clinical findings, a more aggressive approach was elected and a repeat targeted US was performed. US-guided core biopsy was performed, which was positive for invasive carcinoma. An attempted lumpectomy was performed, and final pathology demonstrated a 3.8-cm invasive lobular carcinoma with multiple positive margins.

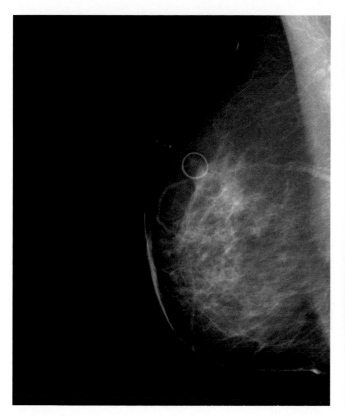

Plate 12.3A

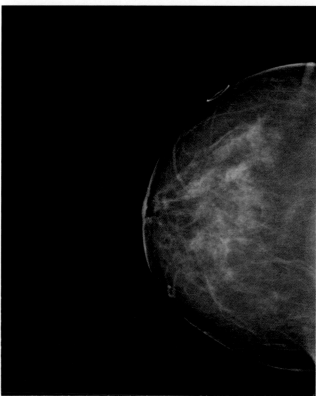

Plate 12.3B

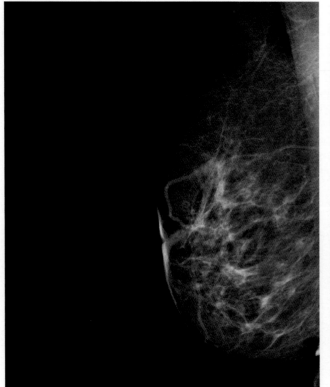

Plate 12.3C

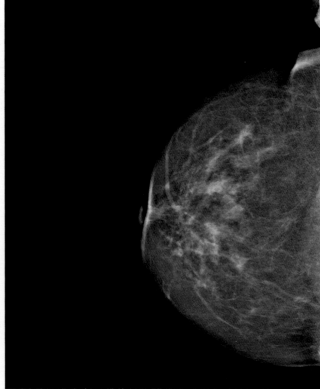

Plate 12.3D

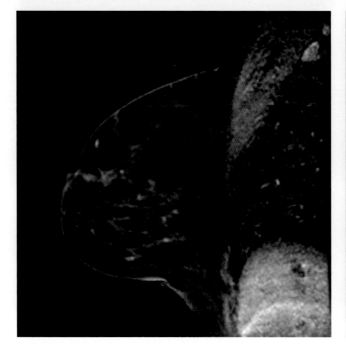

Plate 12.3E

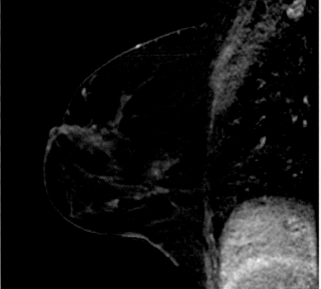

Plate 12.3F

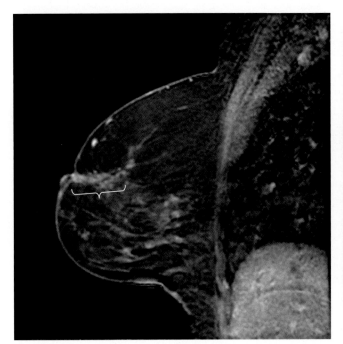

Plate 12.3G

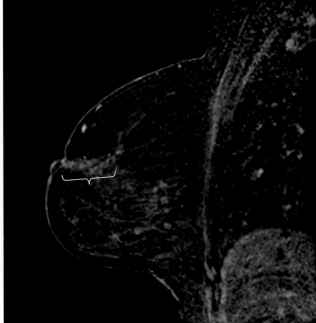

Plate 12.3H

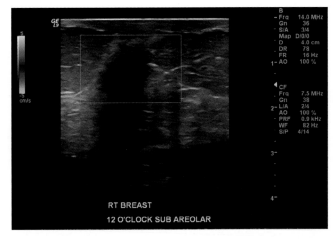

Plate 12.3I

FINDINGS

- Plates 12.3A–B—Mammogram 2 years prior, demonstrating normal breast, no retraction at nipple.
- Plates 12.3C–D—Mammogram with nipple retraction and periareolar skin thickening.
- Plates 12.3E–F—Postcontrast, first series MRI demonstrates the nipple retraction and faint retroareolar-enhancing foci but no mass.
- Plate 12.3G—Last postcontrast series with faint retroareolar enhancement, relatively nonspecific.
- Plate 12.3H—Subtracted fourth postcontrast series demonstrating faint clumped retroareolar enhancement and grouped enhancing foci.
- Plate 12.3I—Targeted US demonstrating the nipple with retroareolar shadowing.

DISCUSSION

On digital mammography, dermal thickening and periareolar skin retraction is evident. However, on MRI, nipple enhancement is normal, and nipple inversion (benign or malignant) can appear as nodular enhancing area in the direct retroareolar region. In a patient with new nipple inversion, this finding should not be ignored. In this case, there was very low level enhancement, but mammographic and clinical changes were severe. The less suspicious MRI findings should not preclude the usual follow-up you would recommend for abnormal mammographic/sonographic/clinical findings. Do not use a negative MRI to supersede the recommendations generated by clinical and other imaging findings. In this case, the lesion was underestimated on MRI, and the ultimate size of the lesion was a surprise at the time of surgery. Invasive lobular carcinoma may fail to enhance or enhance only faintly and slowly and is, therefore, a source of false negative MRI. While this case is not completely negative on MRI, it is easy to see how this kind of malignancy can be missed, especially if there is significant background enhancement.

• Plate 4

HISTORY

A 55-year-old woman with positive family history and digital mammography complicated by extremely dense breast parenchyma and innumerable calcifications. Right upper outer quadrant calcifications were thought to have increased and stereotactic biopsy was performed. Pathology demonstrated atypia. MRI was performed and demonstrated severe enhancement and innumerable bilateral enhancing foci and nodules for which a 6-month follow-up MRI was recommended. Right excisional breast biopsy demonstrated atypical lobular and ductal hyperplasia. She opted for bilateral prophylactic mastectomy. Final pathology demonstrated an incidental 1.1-cm invasive mucinous/colloid carcinoma on the right (inner upper quadrant) and a 0.4-cm low-grade DCIS on left.

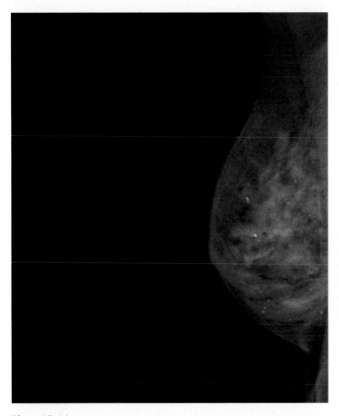

Plate 12.4A

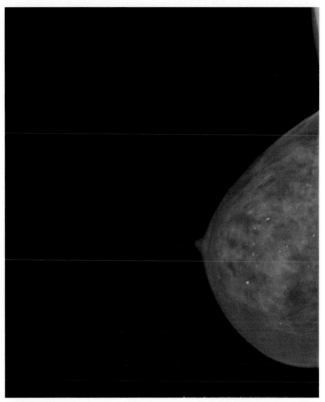

Plate 12.4B

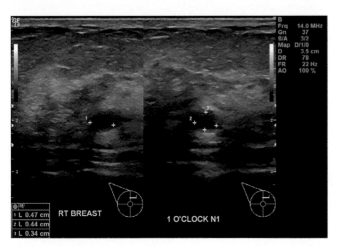

Plate 12.4C

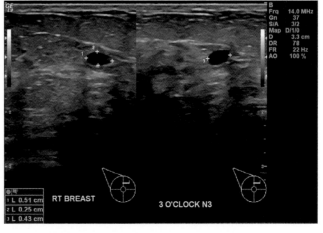

Plate 12.4D

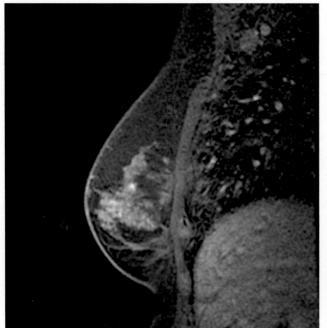

Plate 12.4E

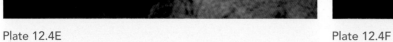

Plate 12.4F

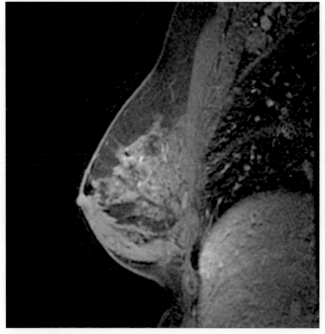

Plate 12.4G

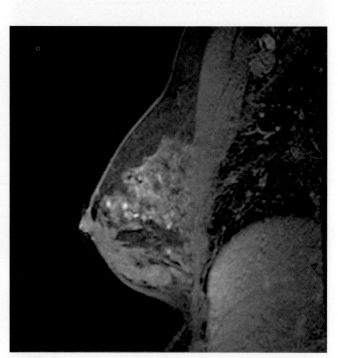

Plate 12.4H

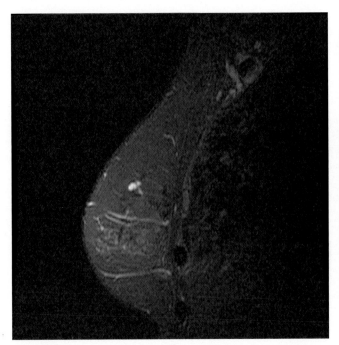

Plate 12.4I

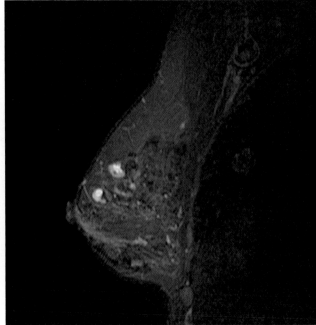

Plate 12.4J

FINDINGS

- Plates 12.4A–B—Right breast mammogram, which demonstrates extremely dense breast parenchyma, numerous calcifications, and a clip from previous stereotactic biopsy.
- Plates 12.4C–D—US demonstrating multiple simple and complex cysts.
- Plates 12.4E–J—MRI. Postcontrast sagittal images through right inner breast, demonstrating innumerable areas of clumped nodular and stippled enhancement thought to be likely glandular. No focal area was more suspicious than the remaining areas.
- Plates 12.4J–I—Sagittal stir images demonstrating high signal lesions thought to represent cysts in the right upper inner quadrant.

DISCUSSION

This 1.1-cm carcinoma was not detected on MRI. There were extensive bilateral enhancing nodular areas, which probably corresponded to areas of atypical lobular and ductal hyperplasia. In addition, there is severe glandular/fibrocystic background enhancement, which also limits the sensitivity of MRI. The final pathology demonstrated a mucinous carcinoma, composed almost entirely of mucin. These lesions are bright on T2/STIR imaging and can enhance the way a cyst does (rim only) when there is little solid component. On the left side, the small focus of low-grade DCIS would be obscured by the background of extreme glandular enhancement. Differentiating a cyst from a mucinous carcinoma with minimal solid component is difficult. Check the smoothness of the inner and outer margin of the enhancing rim around the cyst, and be more suspicious if either of these is irregular. Although this probably suggests inflammation, it can also indicate the presence of a cystic or mucinous carcinoma. If noted, consider targeted US and aspiration/biopsy. Findings that are very high intensity on sagittal STIRS include cysts, lymph nodes and some fibroadenomas. However, since mucinous/colloid carcinomas are also usually high signal on STIRS, you cannot disregard any enhancement of these structures.

• Plate 5

HISTORY

An 83-year-old woman presents with a hypoechoic nodule on US. A needle core biopsy was performed and demonstrated atypical cells. An MRI scan was performed as part of her preoperative evaluation and demonstrated bilateral multiple enhancing foci and small nodules. This amount of background enhancement is unusual in this age group unless the patient is taking hormone replacement therapy. In this woman, there was a history of alcohol abuse, which may also affect hormone levels and background enhancement. No lesion is seen at the biopsy site on MRI. Subsequent localization and biopsy demonstrated a 6-mm apocrine-type DCIS. Papillomatosis and atypia were also present.

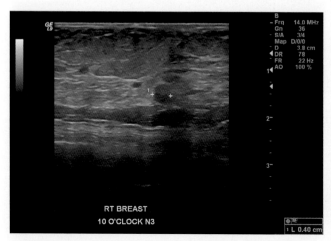

Plate 12.5A

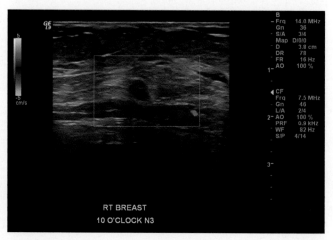

Plate 12.5B

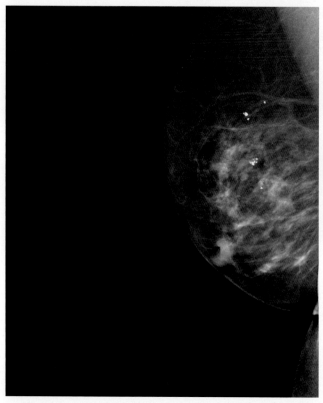

Plate 12.5C

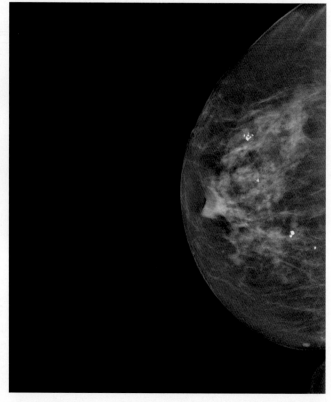

Plate 12.5D

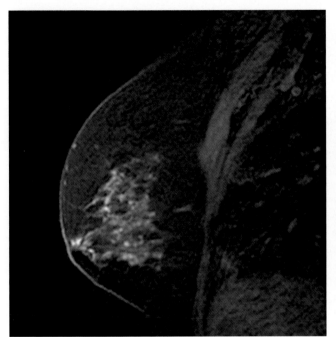

Plate 12.5E

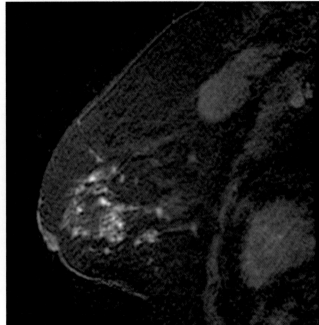

Plate 12.5F

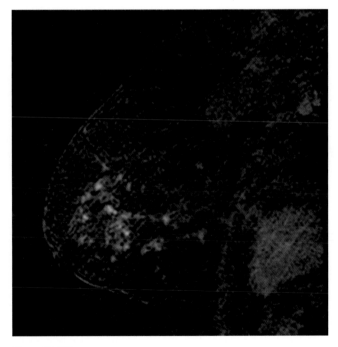

Plate 12.5G

FINDINGS

- Plates 12.5A–B—US demonstrating a hypoechoic nodule with a slightly lobulated margin.
- Plates 12.5C–D—Postbiopsy digital mammography demonstrating clip at site of hypoechoic nodule. Heterogeneously dense parenchyma & benign appearing calcifications are noted.
- Plates 12.5E–G—Selected MRI postcontrast and subtracted images demonstrating innumerable enhancing foci.

DISCUSSION

In this case, the lesion is very small, which makes it more likely to be missed. In addition, the low-grade nature of the DCIS may make it less likely to enhance (although as stated earlier in this text, we have not found failure to enhance to reliably predict that an area of DCIS is low grade). The background enhancement from alcohol abuse can obscure findings the way it would for someone on hormone replacement. In these patients, MRI can be less sensitive.

Since MRI is performed in sections, tiny lesions are easily missed. If you are using a slice thickness of approximately 2.5 mm, you can easily miss a 3-mm lesion, especially when there is any component of patient motion.

Although MRI is more sensitive for detection of breast cancer the spatial resolution of mammographic images is much higher. Again, do *not* disregard indeterminate or suspicious mammographic or sonographic findings simply because you cannot find a corresponding abnormality on MRI; this could lead to a delay in diagnosis.

INDEX

Note: Page numbers followed by an "*f*" denote figures; those followed by a "*t*" denote tables and those with **bold** indicate plates.